New Approaches to Family Practice

SAGE SOURCEBOOKS FOR THE HUMAN SERVICES SERIES

Series Editors: ARMAND LAUFFER and CHARLES GARVIN

Recent Volumes in This Series

HEALTH PROMOTION AT THE COMMUNITY LEVEL
edited by NEIL BRACHT

ELDER CARE: Family Training and Support
by AMANDA SMITH BARUSCH

SOCIAL WORK PRACTICE WITH ASIAN AMERICANS
edited by SHARLENE MAEDA FURUTO, RENUKA BISWAS, DOUGLAS K.CHUNG, KENJI MURASE, & FARIYAL ROSS-SHERIFF

FAMILY POLICIES AND FAMILY WELL-BEING: The Role of Political Culture
by SHIRLEY L. ZIMMERMAN

FAMILY THERAPY WITH THE ELDERLY
by ELIZABETH R. NEIDHARDT & JO ANN ALLEN

EFFECTIVELY MANAGING HUMAN SERVICE ORGANIZATIONS
by RALPH BRODY

SINGLE-PARENT FAMILIES
by KRIS KISSMAN & JO ANN ALLEN

SUBSTANCE ABUSE TREATMENT: A Family Systems Perspective
edited by EDITH M. FREEMAN

SOCIAL COGNITION AND INDIVIDUAL CHANGE: Current Theory and Counseling Guidelines
by AARON M. BROWER & PAULA S. NURIUS

UNDERSTANDING AND TREATING ADOLESCENT SUBSTANCE ABUSE
by PHILIP P. MUISENER

EFFECTIVE EMPLOYEE ASSISTANCE PROGRAMS: A Guide for EAP Counselors and Managers
by GLORIA CUNNINGHAM

COUNSELING THE ADOLESCENT SUBSTANCE ABUSER: School-Based Intervention and Prevention
by MARLENE MIZIKER GONET

TASK GROUPS IN THE SOCIAL SERVICES
by MARIAN FATOUT & STEVEN R. ROSE

WHAT ABOUT AMERICA'S HOMELESS CHILDREN? Hide and Seek
by PAUL G. SHANE

NEW APPROACHES TO FAMILY PRACTICE: Confronting Economic Stress
by NANCY R. VOSLER

New Approaches to Family Practice

Confronting Economic Stress

Nancy R. Vosler

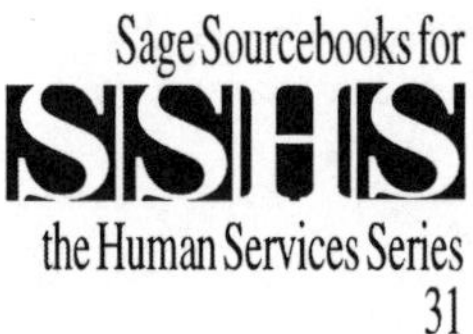

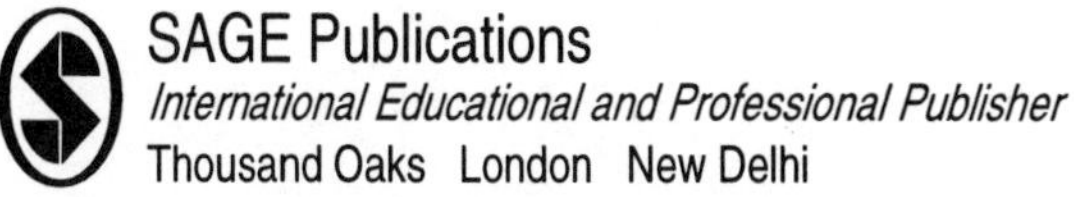

For information address:

SAGE Publications, Inc.
2455 Teller Road
Thousand Oaks, California 91320
E-mail: order@sagepub.com

Sage Publications Ltd.
6 Bonhill Street
London EC2A 4PU
United Kingdom

Sage Publications India Pvt. Ltd.
M-32 Market
Greater Kailash I
New Delhi 110 048 India

Printed in the United States of America

Library of Congress Cataloging-in-Publication Data

Vosler, Nancy R.
New approaches to family practice: confronting economic stress / Nancy R. Vosler.
p. cm. — (Sage sourcebooks for the human services; vol. 31)
Includes bibliographical references (p.) and index.
ISBN 0-7619-0032-2 (cloth: acid-free paper). — ISBN 0-7619-0033-0 (pbk.: acid-free paper)
1. Family social work. 2. Social work with the unemployed. 3. Poor—Services for. 4. Family—Economic aspects. 5. Work and the human services series; v. 31.
HV697.V67 1996
362.82′8—dc20 96-10083

96 97 98 99 00 10 9 8 7 6 5 4 3 2 1

Sage Production Editor: Michèle Lingre

CONTENTS

LIST OF FIGURES

PREFACE

After searching for a number of years for a family practice text that directly addresses social work with families confronting issues of poverty, unemployment, and work-related stress, I finally decided to write this book. I will be using it in my masters'-level theory for practice family course at the George Warren Brown School of Social Work at Washington University in St. Louis. I am confident that it can be used equally well as a text in MSW foundation-level practice overview courses, in family-focused human behavior courses, in advanced family practice courses, and in human behavior and practice courses at the undergraduate level. In addition, concepts and summaries of literature should be useful in applied non-social-work courses dealing with the family. The theoretical material has already been successfully used outside of the United States in a training course for family service staff in Asia.

The core impetus for writing the book came from the realization that a basic assumption of current family systems practice—including family therapy and family preservation models—is flawed. The flawed assumption is "If the family system changes, [all] significant problems can be resolved." Having worked in the child welfare and juvenile justice systems in inner-city urban neighborhoods for a number of years, I know from experience that high unemployment, poverty, poor housing, crime, and lack of accessible services create barriers to effective work with both individuals and families. I've often said that in my quest for understanding effective direct practice, I have been driven to consider macro systems and structures.

When I returned to formal schooling in 1980—with the career goal of earning a PhD for teaching social work—I had the opportunity to immerse myself in two very exciting sets of literature: (a) systemic family therapy models—Bowen, Haley, Minuchin, Satir, and others—and (b) social science-based family studies—arising in large measure from the work of members of the National Council on Family Relations (NCFR) and NCFR publications, *Journal of Marriage and the Family, Family Relations,* and *Journal of Family Issues.* Since the early 1980s, I have taught family theory and practice courses on a regular basis. I have for a long time been frustrated, however, with how to teach a course that combines material from these two sets of literature and what text or combinations of texts to use. Such books as Hartman and Laird's (1983) *Family-Centered Social Work Practice,* Carter and McGoldrick's (1988) *The Changing Family Life Cycle,* and Walsh's (1993) *Normal Family Processes* are excellent sources for teaching students to think about family systems as well as to begin to assess problems and patterns for the purpose of planning interventions. But the "family therapy" approach to family practice seems to assume that services and structures necessary for healthy family functioning are in place and simply need to be accessed and mobilized by the family or the clinician. In this regard, it is perhaps crucial to note that a number of the family therapy models were developed out of work with white middle-class families who indeed often do have access to essential economic and service resources—resources that I am convinced must be developed for all families in our many demographically varied and rapidly changing societies across the globe.

Some family practice authors—notably Bowen, Minuchin, Boyd-Franklin, and others—have called attention to the impact of intersystem conflicts in larger systems on the problems and patterns seen in troubled families and have noted the need for cooperation among professionals and coordination of services. The theoretical connections to changes in larger systems—particularly economic changes resulting in work stress, unemployment, and increasing poverty, detailed by family-oriented social science research studies—have not been highlighted or adequately incorporated into family practice models, however.

Thus, I argue in this book that both *thinking* about problems and, especially, *targeting* interventions must increasingly become "multilevel"—that is, focused not on family systems alone but equally on neighborhoods and local communities, and on policies and structures at state, national, and global levels. I present and discuss case examples of effective new practice approaches and delineate tools for multilevel assessment and intervention.

In my courses, I will certainly continue to use other texts in conjunction with this book—including both the NCFR decade reviews of family research and family practice classics. But I am convinced that in the ongoing social, economic, political, and cultural changes in the United States, to practice effectively, social workers and other human service professionals must be able to conceptualize their direct practice work within an understanding of larger systems and structures and of needed change. Just as the family therapy movement gave birth to the shift from focusing exclusively on treating the individual to "seeing" the person in the context of family patterns and needed changes, so must social workers and other human service professionals now work to shift both their own and fellow citizens' thinking from an exclusive focus on "fixing" families—to seeing individuals and families in the context of larger systems and necessary *multilevel* change. If this book contributes to a shift in current thinking in family practice toward incorporating this multilevel approach, I'll consider the endeavor a success.

ACKNOWLEDGMENTS

This book has been "a long time coming" and would not have been possible without the help, support, and encouragement of many, many people.

Robert Green at Virginia Commonwealth University School of Social Work introduced me to family systems thinking and simultaneously to the importance of theory and empirical research for practice knowledge development. He also read and commented extensively on a first draft of the manuscript and encouraged me to complete the project. Others who especially nurtured my early learning regarding families and knowledge building for practice have included Martin Bloom, Katharine Briar, Anne Fortune, and Ann Hartman.

The community of scholars at the George Warren Brown School of Social Work at Washington University in St. Louis has provided the environment of intellectual challenge and support within which my thinking has developed and come to this stage of fruition. Dean Shanti Khinduka has given encouragement, several faculty research awards, and a sabbatical leave during which I was able to begin the long task of getting ideas onto paper. Faculty colleagues have discussed ideas, read and commented on drafts, and believed the project could be completed. I particularly want to thank Larry Davis, Therese Dent, Shanta Pandey, Enola Proctor, Mark Rank, Michael Sherraden, and Gautam Yadama.

Washington University MSW, PhD, and undergraduate students, in classes and individually, have helped to shape my questions and ideas. Then-PhD-student Deborah Page-Adams collaborated on an unemployment research project and read and commented on a draft of chapters. Cynthia Rocha and I had long conversations about families and poverty. MSW students Pamela Fitch, Karen Krischker, and Jennifer Johnson assisted with literature searches; Shirley Crenshaw read a draft and made very helpful suggestions.

My thinking has also been profoundly influenced by opportunities for collaboration with practitioners both in St. Louis and in Singapore. Jean Caine read an early draft and encouraged me to continue with the project. Janice Olson of Provident Counseling provided invaluable suggestions and detailed feedback on the manuscript. In Singapore, collaboration with Sudha Nair, Myrna Blake, Pang Kee Tai, Suraya, Ng Guat Tin, and others at The Ang Mo Kio Family Service Centres allowed me to reflect on both family diversity and common human realities.

Production of the manuscript would not have been possible without the support of David Cronin, and the able and patient assistance of Vivian Westbrook, Lisa Mathis, Suzanne Fragale, and Jennica Dotseth. I also want to thank Rhonda Winstead for her magical computer work on the graphics.

I deeply appreciate the encouragement and guidance I have received from Series Editor Charles Garvin and from Jim Nageotte at Sage Publications.

Finally, I want to thank my extended families—the Benoits, Days, Rose-Cooks, Roses, Smith-Voslers, Thompsons, and Voslers—for "being there" in my reflections on families and society. Most of all, I want to thank my husband, Mike, for believing from the very beginning that this undertaking was important and doable. His support, encouragement, and optimism in the face of frustrations and inevitable detours have seen me through to the successful completion of this project.

Research for this book was supported by a faculty research award by the George Warren Brown School of Social Work, Washington University, St. Louis.

NANCY R. VOSLER

Chapter 1

INTRODUCTION
Social Work Knowledge Building

In the United States and worldwide, a number of critical controversies focus on families and on negative and positive changes among diverse types of families. Social workers and other human service professionals, including direct service providers, administrators, program and policy practitioners, researchers, educators, and students, require up-to-date knowledge for effective practice.

Increasingly, stresses from economic changes at local, state, national, and even global levels are impacting families. Family stressors resulting from macroeconomic shifts include (a) decreasing wages, increases in dual-earner families, and potential role overload in both employed work and family work; (b) loss of high-wage unionized jobs in the manufacturing sector, with subsequent increases in unemployment and underemployment; and (c) increasing poverty, particularly among families with children.

Families struggling with these interrelated stressors are likely to be served by direct service social work practitioners and other human service professionals. Most family practice models focus assessment and change efforts on the family—without clearly assessing the impact of stress from larger social systems on the family's current functioning and without targeting change efforts at larger systems beyond the family. Theoretical development and research studies, particularly in family sociology, have begun to provide empirically based knowledge regarding macroeconomic issues and their correlates and consequences for families; application of this theoretical knowledge via models for multilevel social work practice requires expansion of current—and development of new—knowledge for practice.

My overall aim in this book is to contribute to family practice knowledge-development efforts. One aspect of this enterprise is the provision of an overview of current social science theory and empirical findings regarding families and family issues. Three specific areas are particularly relevant to social work practice with families experiencing stress from larger environments: (a) macroeconomic changes and their impact on *employed work and family work* in families, (b) *unemployment* and its impact on family functioning, and (c) *poverty* and its impact on family members as well as on the formation and dissolution of families. My focus in this literature review is to link research to *practice*. In addition, I explore ways for social work practitioners—especially direct service social workers—to clearly grasp that they have important and usable empirical information that is critical in understanding families and their difficulties. Such information must become part of the development of innovations for working with stressed families to achieve healthy functioning within supportive larger social systems.

As context for discussion of this material and its implications for professional knowledge building and practice, in this chapter I address three interrelated topics: (a) the relationship between social work practice and empirical research; (b) social science theory and research, with a specific focus on families; and (c) social work knowledge building for guiding professional practice with and on behalf of families. In the final section of this chapter, I delineate for readers the organizational structure of the book.

SOCIAL WORK PRACTICE AND EMPIRICAL RESEARCH

Debate continues regarding the exact role of empirical research in social work practice (Dunlap, 1993) and over whether social work research is "applied social science" (Klein & Bloom, 1994). It is clear, however, that social workers interested in family practice have much to learn from and contribute to knowledge building in at least two broad areas: (a) social research regarding "normal" families and how diverse kinds of families function, and (b) studies that focus on issues and problems that families face and on innovative interventions and solu-

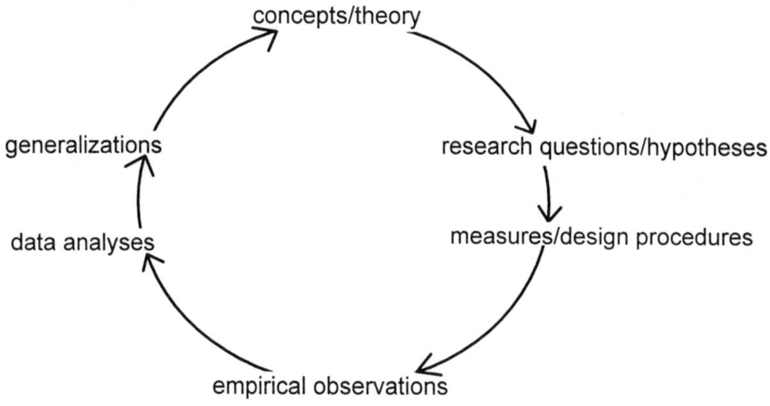

Figure 1.1. Social Science Theory Building

tions. Thus, as noted by Garvin and Seabury (1984), propositional knowledge (describing populations, contexts, problems, etc.) and procedural knowledge (derived from evaluations of specific interventions and procedures) are both needed for continuous social work theory building for effective practice (Proctor, Davis, & Vosler, 1995).

Research methods are procedures for "knowing" reality and are avenues for social workers' participation in communities of scholars engaged in broad-based and ongoing knowledge development. The underlying process of social science theory building is summarized in Figure 1.1. In this view, knowledge emerges not just from theorizing or observation but from a continuous process of constructing theory, developing research questions or testable hypotheses, generating data from empirical observations, organizing these data into generalizations, linking these generalizations back into theory, and continuing the process, either to replicate the previous results or to modify the initial research questions or hypotheses. In this process, there are no clear beginning or end points. Knowledge building is an ongoing enterprise (Rubin & Babbie, 1993).

A variety of research methods have been created for developing knowledge. These include both quantitative and qualitative methods and a variety of designs. Designs include field research, content analysis, historical research, comparative research, survey research, evaluation research, use of existing data, and experiments. (For further discussion, see Babbie, 1992.) Quantitative methods—such as surveys and use of existing statistics—can provide descriptions of broad populations. Studies based on these methods "emphasize the production of precise and generalizable statistical findings" (Rubin & Babbie, 1993, p. 30). Alternatively, qualitative methods such as case studies, participant observation, informal and open-ended interviews, and analysis of historical information provide richer but less generalizable findings.

Some recent family research has combined both quantitative and qualitative methods in important and creative ways. For example, Rank (1994), in his study of welfare recipients, entitled *Living on the Edge: The Realities of Welfare in America,* has utilized a variety of qualitative and quantitative data.

Paradigms or theoretical frameworks are critical components of the research process. Rubin and Babbie (1993) define a paradigm as "a fundamental model or scheme that organizes our view of something" (p. 45). A number of paradigms are utilized by social workers, including "psychosocial, functionalist, problem-solving, cognitive-behavioral, task-centered, case management, crisis intervention, ecological perspective, life model, generalist, empirically based practice, eclectic, and others" (p. 47). These authors also note, "Although a paradigm doesn't necessarily answer important questions, it tells us where to look for the answers. And . . . where you look largely determines the answers you'll find" (p. 45).

Understanding the paradigms and broad theoretical frameworks being utilized by social scientists and social workers can enhance relationships between disciplines. Constructive critique of paradigms and related methods, findings, and conclusions can lead to effective interdisciplinary dialogue and knowledge development. The primary theoretical frameworks or paradigms used in this book are (a) a multilevel social systems perspective, (b) a family development (family life cycle) framework, (c) a social construction view of social systems, and (d) the stress and coping perspective.

A key to knowledge development is conceptualization, that is, the clear specification of terms. Concepts can sometimes enable social workers to "see" realities that had previously been "invisible." For example, the coining of the term *family work* by Pleck (see Piotrkowski & Hughes, 1993, p. 191) and others has helped to break down the false dichotomy of family versus work (in which "work" means "employed work"). Use of the term family work has resulted in discussion and research regarding the energy, time, and management skills necessary for accomplishment of "the household chores and childcare tasks that must be performed by families to maintain the household and its members" (Piotrkowski & Hughes, 1993, p. 191).

In addition, concepts are key elements for building the theories that are needed to guide the development and evaluation of practice techniques and models. Thus, it is important that key concepts emerge from and be related back to practice if social work research is to be usable by direct service, administrative, and policy practitioners.

Bloom, Wood, and Chambon (1991), in their discussion of "the six languages of social work," note that the "empirical language" of variables and measurement is a key component of social work knowledge building. The six "languages" are (a) the lay language of the client, (b) the abstract language of the theorist, (c) the empirical language of the researcher, (d) the categorical language of the information scientist, (e) the formal language of the helping professional, and (f) the preferential language that conveys values. Critical to the ongoing social work knowledge-building enterprise is the development of measurement tools and procedures. This "translation," or operationalization of abstract concepts into empirical variables, through the development of valid and reliable indicators, measures, and instruments, is a difficult and ongoing set of tasks.

Social workers, because of their commitment to a practice that includes diverse and oppressed populations, have a key role to play in the continuing critique of current measurement tools and instruments. Many standardized research scales and inventories have been normed primarily on white, middle-class U.S. populations and may not be valid for other population groups, such as people of color, ethnic minorities, women, gay men, lesbians, the elderly, families with low income, and persons with disabilities.

Ethical and effective social work practice—including research—must be particularly sensitive to issues of diversity not only in the development of valid assessment and measurement tools but also in the entire knowledge-building enterprise, including the critique of previous research methods, concepts, and theories. In Chapter 3, I address practice (including research) with client families differing ethnically or in other ways from the practitioner. Collaboration and consultation are often critical in understanding particular clients' difficulties and issues.

RESEARCH ON FAMILIES

Social work with families has been an important component of professional practice since Mary Richmond (1917), and social workers have been active contributors to the development of theory and practice models in the family therapy movement. Virginia Satir (1964, 1988), a social worker, was one of the first to conceptualize links to society as an important component for assessment and work with families. Other social workers contributing to ongoing, primarily procedural knowledge development in the interdisciplinary family therapy field include Harry Aponte, Elizabeth Carter, Lynn Hoffman, Monica McGoldrick, Peggy Papp, Olga Silverstein, Froma Walsh, and Marianne Walters, among others (Hartman & Laird, 1987; Proctor et al., 1995). Hartman and Laird's *Family-Centered Social Work Practice* (1983) enhanced social work by establishing an ongoing process of drawing theory and models from the family therapy movement into the mainstream of social work professional practice. Work by Davis and Proctor (1989) has contributed to procedural knowledge building by synthesizing extant empirical research regarding impacts of race, gender, and class on professional practice with families.

Parallel to this procedural knowledge development but often somewhat peripheral to social work research, education, and practice has been a virtual explosion of largely propositional empirical research on many aspects of families and family life. Much of this work has been interdisciplinary in nature, although it initially emerged primarily from the general area of family sociology or "family science." This knowledge development effort has been guided and shaped to a significant degree by the work of members of the National Council on Family Relations (NCFR) and the council's journals, the *Journal of Marriage and the Family* and *Family Relations;* NCFR also sponsors the *Journal of Family Issues.*

Beginning in 1970, NCFR has published "decade reviews" (i.e., in 1970, 1980, and 1990/91) of social science research and theory regarding marriage and the family. Felix Berardo (1980), editor of the 1970-1979 decade review, states,

> In the continual effort to advance our understanding of human behavior, social scientists find it both necessary and useful to make periodic assessments of the accumulated knowledge in their respective disciplines. . . . The contributors to this volume are all active researchers and theoreticians

> in the specialties they have reviewed. They are intimately acquainted with the latest findings and are in a unique position to evaluate the implications of these findings and their contributions to the overall development of the field [of marriage and the family]. . . . It is our hope that this volume will serve a wide range of needs. . . . On a . . . practical and pragmatic level, we foresee the volume serving as a reference and overview for those individuals involved in policymaking and the everyday exigencies of program development and implementation. (p. iii)

Findings from this body of propositional knowledge often are not a central part of social work professional discussion and practice theory development, however, perhaps because these decade reviews are often primarily in the "languages" (Bloom et al., 1991) of theory, research, and information science. Discussions of implications within these reviews tend to focus on future research rather than on "translation" into social work practice models and innovations. This gap between propositional family social science knowledge and social work practice with families must be bridged: The richness of current theory and empirical research regarding families must become a central and dynamic part of the knowledge base of social work (e.g., within the Human Behavior and the Social Environment and Social Work Practice curricula), and social workers must increase their contribution toward developing both propositional and procedural knowledge of effective solutions for interconnected individual, family, and larger social system problems and issues.

To contribute to a process of summarizing, critiquing, and translating existing social science findings into usable social work practice theories, models, and tools, I provide an overview from the 1990 NCFR decade review (Booth, 1991) along with other relevant as well as more recent books and articles. Note that most of the articles in Booth (1991) are also in the November, 1990 issue of the *Journal of Marriage and the Family.* The materials considered here cover three specific areas of family life: (a) family work and employed work, (b) unemployment, and (c) poverty.

KNOWLEDGE BUILDING FOR PRACTICE

Clearly, it is important to ensure that social work practitioners who work with families have ready access to the most up-to-date propositional social science knowledge regarding families and family issues. Of equal and complementary importance is the development of mechanisms whereby direct service providers, administrators, and policy and program practitioners can contribute to ongoing propositional and procedural knowledge-building efforts to achieve effective "family-centered social work practice" (Hartman & Laird, 1983).

Social workers and other human service professionals working with families have a rich array of data and understandings about families' problems and their contexts, and about what works and does not work with particular families and family members. But again using Bloom et al.'s (1991) "six languages" conceptualization, beginning in the 1920s and 1930s, a dichotomy developed in the social work profession (Dunlap, 1993) between the three more practice-oriented languages (professional practice, lay/client, and preferential values) and the three more empirical-research-oriented languages (theory/concepts, empirical research operationalizations, and statistical/mathematical analyses). In addition, the professional practice and theory/concepts languages became split between more individually oriented, "micro" theoretical frameworks and paradigms (e.g., psychodynamic, behavioral/cognitive, and later family systems theories and practice models) and more societally oriented, or "macro" practice techniques and models (e.g., advocacy and lobbying, community organizing, and social development). These separations have resulted in difficulties in communication and a lack of shared bases for cross-language collaborative knowledge building.

The "person-in-environment" paradigm has continued to hold promise, however, and in some instances to provide solid common ground for stabilizing and maintaining constructive dialogue between micro and macro social work practitioners as well as between practitioners and researchers. Based on theoretical and evaluation work from the family therapy field and empirical research and theory from family social science, I argue for the use of a multilevel social systems model—including family life cycle, stress and coping, and "systems as social constructions" concepts—as a critical theoretical framework for developing knowledge for effective social work practice with families.

In a recent review and discussion of research on family practice, Proctor et al. (1995) conclude that for certain problems, "under conditions of rigorous [empirical] testing, methods of family treatment have shown positive—perhaps even impressive—outcomes" (p. 947). They also note, however, "Although little work has been done to evaluate treatment programs for low-income families, whatever studies have been done have suggested limited success. . . . Similarly, there is little evidence of treatment gains in practice with isolated, impoverished, single-parent families" (p. 947). These findings suggest the need for a variety of family intervention models and approaches as well as for increased attention in both practice and research to the impact on families of stress from larger social systems. These authors conclude that just as social workers have contributed significantly to family practice, practitioners need to see that they have important contributions to make to research and professional knowledge building.

Thus, it is likely that effective knowledge building will involve all of the six "actors" implied in Bloom et al.'s (1991) discussion of languages:

1. Clients and other "lay" persons—for example, participants in services, as coevaluators of programs, supportive neighbors of service users, informed advocates, and voters
2. A variety of professional social workers in both micro and macro roles
3. Researchers and practitioners collaborating in the development of clear concepts and relevant and usable theories
4. Social work practitioners and researchers with expertise in operationalization; measurement; and the use and critique of current measures and techniques, measurement instruments, methods, and designs
5. Researchers who have expertise in mathematical models, statistical packages, and the use of computers and computer software in the analysis of data and who understand the interpretation (and limitations) of statistical results
6. Professionals in a variety of these five roles who share common values and commitments to ethical knowledge development for effective social work practice with and on behalf of families.

Such a knowledge-building effort will require collaboration and dialogue among multiple actors, for seldom does any one person have advanced expertise in all of the languages of social work. In addition, there is much for social workers to learn *from* and contribute *to* a variety of interdisciplinary social science and applied social science efforts (Cheung, 1990). This includes cumulative knowledge building regarding families in the fields of psychology, sociology, anthropology, political science, and economics, and in such applied areas as education, health and mental health, child welfare, juvenile justice, gerontology, urban planning, community development, unemployment, and poverty.

The purpose of this book is to contribute to expanding knowledge. Incorporating multilevel social systems theory into an ongoing research-from-practice/research-for-practice agenda, such knowledge building over time will bring together social work practitioners and researchers along with other social scientists, political leaders, and ordinary citizens—including clients—for discussion and dialogue for furthering the development of substantive and usable theories and knowledge about families and family problems. Equally critical, the wide and continuing dissemination and use of this emerging knowledge will result in discovery of innovative solutions to critical and often seemingly intractable difficulties facing families in the United States and the world.

ORGANIZATION OF THE BOOK

In keeping with the discussion thus far, the organization of the remainder of this book involves two overlapping structural components. The first component, discussed in Chapters 2 and 3, consists of an *overview* of theoretical frameworks regarding families as social systems, with application of this perspective to social work practice with client families. *Summaries* of theories and specific empirical research findings follow as they apply to work with families in *three specific problem areas* that are increasingly affecting U.S. families: role overload from employed work and family work (Chapters 4 and 5), unemployment (Chapters 6 and 7), and poverty (Chapters 8 and 9).

The second structural component is focused on summarizing and linking *empirical theory and research* in Chapters 2, 4, 6, and 8 with the more specific *practice applications and tools* for family-centered social work in Chapters 3, 5, 7, and 9. In Chapter 10, I discuss overall conclusions and implications.

In summary, my goal is (a) to present concepts, theories, and research findings in a language that social work practitioners can use, with an eye to their reciprocation in ongoing knowledge development efforts; and, concomitantly, (b) to identify assessment tools, intervention procedures, and strategies for use in collaborative empirical data gathering and evaluation. The need is for continuing knowledge building by social work researchers and practitioners at both micro and macro social systems levels. We turn now to consideration of a *systemic,* or *social systems,* view of families and of their functioning and problems.

Chapter 2

FAMILY SYSTEMS IN CONTEXT
The Multilevel Social Systems Model

In the past few decades, the systemic or social systems approach has emerged as an important theoretical perspective for understanding and working with families (Anderson & Carter, 1990; Becvar & Becvar, 1993; Broderick, 1993; for general system theory, see Bertalanffy, 1968). This framework is related to social work's person-in-environment, or ecological, perspective (Germain & Gitterman, 1987; for human ecology theory, see Bronfenbrenner, 1979). According to social systems theory, each family is not just a collection of individual members but an organized group of interacting persons who develop roles, rules, beliefs, patterns of communication, and organizational structures for task accomplishment and functioning.

A social systems view involves describing the family as part of and nested in a series of larger systems that likewise develop organizational structures, roles, rules, beliefs, and patterns of communication. These multiple systems levels include the neighborhood, the local community, state and national systems, and the global socioeconomic and ecological systems. At times, families may find these larger systemic structures supportive of family functioning, but these larger systems are organized in ways that deprive some families and their members of resources that are vital for healthy development.

A key concept in the social worker's use of the systemic view is an understanding that social systems are social constructions. According to this perspective, beliefs, patterns, and structures are developed over time by members of the social system. Thus, the organizational structures currently maintained by a family, neighborhood, local, state, or national social system are learned patterns and behaviors. A corollary of this understanding is that change is always possible. If patterns have been learned, they can be unlearned and something new can be learned in their place.

This does not mean that change is simple or easy, for systems tend to maintain an equilibrium or "steady state" (Anderson & Carter, 1990) of old, familiar patterns and structures. Many practitioners who work with distressed families are acutely aware of the powerful tendencies of family systems to maintain painful but familiar ways of functioning. Similarly, neighborhoods—or nations for that matter—do not often easily and quickly achieve radical change to stable new structures. The liberating power of a social construction point of view is that current dysfunctional patterns—which were previously functional, that is, the system's "best solution" at the time—can now be changed with understanding and hard work by system members' striving together to put in place different, more functional patterns.

DEFINITIONS OF FAMILY

As discussed in Chapter 1, concepts and their definitions are a critical component of social science and social work knowledge building. The definition of *family* used by a social work practitioner or researcher consciously or unconsciously shapes the understanding he or she has of practice and of research. For example, a researcher who uses a narrow and rigid "traditional" view of the family as a group of persons related by "a legal, lifelong, sexually exclusive marriage between one man and one woman, with children, where the male is the primary provider and ultimate authority" (Macklin, 1980, p. 175; see, e.g., Parsons & Bales, 1955), will be restricted by this definition in his or her data gathering to a limited number of "familial" groupings within our complex and global society.

A broader, but still fairly traditional, definition is provided by *The Social Work Dictionary,* in which family is defined as "a primary group" based on "blood, adoption, or marriage" (Barker, 1987, p. 53). It should be noted that use of this definition by a practitioner or researcher would exclude lesbian and gay couples and their children who are living together as family. In the past, some child welfare practitioners have been blinded by such limited views of family and have overlooked or ignored African American extended-family households that included "fictive kin" (Martin & Martin, 1985), as well as American Indian tribal relationships that operate as family but are not limited to "blood, adoption, or marriage" (see, e.g., Unger, 1977). As Hartman and Laird (1987, p. 576) have noted, how we define family has important implications not only for direct practice with families but also for how policies and programs at agency, local, state, and national levels frame eligibility for numerous social services (see also Hartman, 1995.)

The definition that will be used in this book is from the 1981 National Association of Social Workers (NASW) Family Policy Statement in which family is defined as "a grouping that consists of two or more individuals who define themselves as a family and who over time assume those obligations to one another that are generally considered an essential component of family systems" (NASW, 1982, p. 10). This self-defined, phenomenological view of family allows the inclusion of a diversity of emerging family forms, including lesbian and gay families, varying extended-family households, and women as heads of families. In addition, implied in the definition is the understanding outlined by Hartman and Laird (1987) that a family "is created when two or more people construct an intimate environment that they define as a family, an environment in which they generally will share a living space, commitment, and a variety of the roles and functions usually considered part of family life" (p. 576).

As will be discussed later in this chapter, a family systems approach that includes a family life cycle view presents social work and other human service professionals with a complex understanding of families. Thus, one's family does not end with one's "family-of-origin" or "growing-up" family, which may include biologically related members as well as adoptive and foster members, and a variety of other familial relationships. For many, there is also a "family-of-procreation" or "decisional" family, which may include one or more partners, children—biological, adopted, fostered, and otherwise related—and possibly, in a remarriage family, other more indirect relationships (for example, a visiting stepchild's custodial parent and grandparents).

Family is a rich and complex concept, involving many important relationships. It is clear that social work with families must be based on an understanding of these relationships that provides a broad and encompassing view of the critical institution of family in our global society.

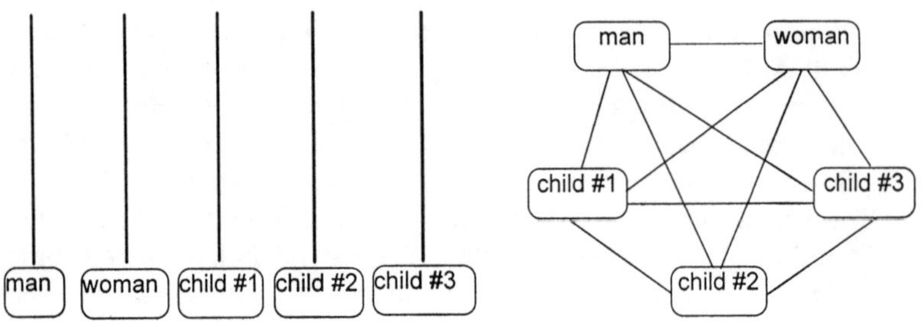

Figure 2.1. The Family As Social System

THE FAMILY AS SOCIAL SYSTEM

A social systems approach to understanding and working with families requires a shift from focusing on particular family members as individuals to attending to relationships and interactional patterns between and among the persons who make up the focal family unit. As illustrated in Figure 2.1, systemic work with families shifts from a one-by-one focus on family members (man, woman, child #1, child #2, etc.) to a focus on tracking the patterns of interrelationship between members of the family or household (husband-wife, father-child #1, mother-father, child #1-mother, child #1-child #2, mother-child #3, etc.). Understanding of dyads and triads (e.g., mother-father-child #3) in the family unit becomes an important focus for attention and possible intervention. The person is seen as nested within a *family system* of relationships that are at least as important for social work and human service knowledge building and practice as are *individual* functioning and problems.

Delineating a working understanding of families as social systems involves several interrelated aspects of this theoretical perspective. In this section,

1. An overview of *key systems concepts* will be presented.
2. System *boundaries and cohesion* will be discussed.
3. Family *organizational structures and roles* will be delineated.

4. An emerging understanding of how family *beliefs and rules* organize and contribute to family life will be discussed.
5. The concept of *communication* in families will be reviewed.
6. The developmental concept of *family life cycle(s)* will be presented and critiqued.

Key Systems Concepts

In an early discussion of family systems theory for clinical practice, Walsh (1982, pp. 9-10) summarized seven general systems principles that distinguish social systems thinking from individualistic approaches: (a) circular causality, (b) nonsummativity, (c) equifinality, (d) communication, (e) family rules, (f) homeostasis, and (g) morphogenesis.

Briefly, *circular causality* refers to sequences of interaction between family members, such that a change in one part of the system affects and is affected by resulting changes in other parts of the system in "a circular chain of influence" (Walsh, 1982, p. 9). A family is metaphorically like a hanging mobile that reacts to a wind gust not as individualistic parts, but as a whole. *Nonsummativity* points to an understanding of family as more than simply a sum of its individual parts (e.g., mother, father, adolescent son), in that differing organizational patterns (rules, beliefs, styles of communication) can result in very different outcomes for family members and the family as a whole. *Equifinality* refers to the fact that in interactional systems, the same initial condition or event (e.g., the birth of a Downs syndrome child) can result in very different family outcomes (e.g., increased cohesion versus divorce of the parents), and the same outcome (a single-parent household) may flow from a variety of origins (death of a parent, divorce, parents never married).

Walsh (1982, p. 10) notes that from a family systems perspective, *communication* encompasses all interpersonal behaviors both verbal and nonverbal, and that clear communication is essential for healthy system functioning. *Family rules* are patterned and predictable norms or expectations that explicitly or implicitly govern behavior and relationships in the family; they can be observed in repetitious sequences of interaction between family members.

Homeostasis and *morphogenesis* are a pair of concepts used to describe stability and change in family systems. Homeostasis refers to the tendency of social systems "to maintain a steady, stable state in the ongoing interaction system" (Walsh, 1982, p. 10), using positive or negative reinforcing feedback loops to regulate or restore the current organizational equilibrium. Morphogenesis refers to "second-order change" (p. 10) that involves a shift or reorganization of family rules and patterns, often in response to changes in external systems, or involving internal family life cycle transitions. Substantial shifts in role allocations (e.g., household maintenance and child care) resulting from a stay-at-home mother reentering the labor force following the closing of the auto manufacturing plant where her husband has worked for 10 years is an example of morphogenetic change. These two concepts are particularly critical for social work family researchers and practitioners, as an understanding of the dynamics of both stability and needed change is necessary for effective work with distressed families.

Boundaries and Cohesion

Important concepts in assessment of families are family boundaries and cohesion. Boundary questions of who is included in a focal family unit and who is not can be defined by family members. Some researchers have used a "household" (Popenoe, 1993) view of the family, that is, all members living under the same roof over time. Others have focused on legal boundaries involving biological kinship, marriage, or adoption. A recent discussion of divorced families suggests a "pedifocal" definition, which includes community members—including child care providers—and fictive kin who have "status and role responsibilities in the family" related to child rearing (Crosbie-Burnett & Lewis, 1993, p. 244). In practice, discussions with the family about whom to include in change efforts can reveal for both the worker and family members patterns of inclusion and exclusion between various members of the family network.

In addition, concepts from family life cycle theory illuminate the fact that family boundaries develop and change over time. A newly married young couple may draw the boundaries tightly around their new family, wanting to establish autonomy and distance from their respective families of origin. In addition, intrafamily boundaries for individual autonomy are important within the family unit. Beavers (1982), for example, delineates the importance of "closeness" that includes *both* connection *and* distinct boundaries (see also Beavers & Hampson, 1993). The McMaster Model of Family Functioning similarly emphasizes the importance of connection (affective responsiveness and involvement) and similarly cautions against overinvolvement ("symbiotic involvement") (Epstein, Bishop, & Baldwin, 1982).

On the other hand, many newly established families in various cultures around the world do not have the choice of financial independence and may live within a parental home for a time after the marriage. Even where couples live in extended-family households, however, it is often important for the newly formed family to establish emotional boundaries for intimacy and decision making.

In addition, a life cycle understanding alerts researchers and practitioners to the possibility that as children are born, extended-family members may participate in child care, especially when both parents work outside the home, resulting in an increased connection with grandparents or other relatives. As children grow into adolescence, internal and external family boundaries often need modification to meet changing needs of family members for intrafamily cohesion and closeness as well as for autonomy and extrafamilial relationships and peer friendships. As grandparents age, there may be a need for increased connection or even physical inclusion in the household to assure adequate care.

Decisions about whom to include as members in the focal family unit will need to be made to understand and work with a particular family. Equally important is an understanding of the history and quality of family connections and boundaries that have preceded this mutually defined family unit.

Building on the concept of boundaries, Satir (1988) emphasized the importance of understanding the degree to which systems are closed or open. Closed systems tend to become rigid and dysfunctionally isolated from the larger society, whereas open systems are more able to adapt in healthy response to change in both external systems and individual members' development. Similarly, Olson, Sprenkle, and Russell (1979) have conceptualized "family cohesion" on a continuum, with variable healthy styles of "separated" or "connected" in a balanced middle and dysfunctional styles of "disengaged" or "enmeshed" at the extremes (see also Olson, 1993; Olson & Lavee, 1989; Thomas & Olson, 1993). All of these conceptualizations converge on the need for connectedness and closeness, but with clear boundaries that provide emotional "space" for diversity, individuality, and change.

Organizational Structures and Roles

Family systems exhibit organization-like structures and roles. Anderson and Carter (1990) define role as "a set of expectations regarding behavior that can be fulfilled by a person . . . ;[these] expectations

. . . are defined and sanctioned by significant environmental systems" (p. 265). Structures are "the most stable relationships between systems and components (i.e., with the slowest rate of change)" (p. 266). An important perspective from which to analyze family systems is as a small ongoing organization with specific sets of roles and organizational structures for carrying out tasks and functions in the larger society.

The primary functions of families (identified by Lewis, Beavers, Gossett, & Phillips, 1976) are the nurturance of adult family members and the raising of the next generation. For these functions to be carried out, responsibility for various roles must be allocated and structures for accountability developed (Epstein et al., 1982). Role allocation and accountability structures include basic provision, leadership and decision making, household maintenance, dependents' care, and child rearing and socialization. Family role allocation has shifted in the past several decades, often in response to economic and political changes in larger systems. The content and importance of each area will be briefly delineated here.

A critical set of tasks in every family is the *provision* of basic resources for survival of members, including adequate food, shelter, clothing, and medical care. Successful performance of the provider role in complex capitalist industrial societies depends to some extent on larger systems' organization of employment and wages, as they link with affordable housing and utilities, appropriate personal and household goods, and such services as health care. Recent research regarding these issues is examined in detail in Chapters 4, 6, and 8.

A second important set of roles is *leadership and decision making* in the family unit. This set of tasks has been identified as critical by a number of theorists, focusing on the importance of a parental alliance and hierarchy (e.g., Haley, Minuchin, etc.; see Walsh, 1982), shared power (Beavers, 1982), appropriate discipline (Thomas & Olson, 1993), and behavior control (Epstein et al., 1982).

The tasks of *household maintenance and management* are repetitious and seemingly ordinary but important and often time-consuming activities. They include shopping, cooking, washing dishes, cleaning, doing laundry, repairing appliances, doing (or arranging for) household repairs, yard work, and so forth. Management also involves arranging for family members to get to and from activities and appointments, planning family outings and celebrations, and creating spaces and times for friends to visit. All of this is often taken for granted by family members and the larger society, but the successful performance of these roles and tasks requires both knowledge and skill.

The *care of dependents* as an important set of family tasks and roles has seen renewed focus and discussion in recent years as the proportion of elderly in industrialized societies has increased. This care includes not only frail elderly parents but also children and sick and disabled family members.

Separate from, but related to, physical care of dependent children are the critical roles and tasks of *rearing children and youth.* This includes their individual cognitive and affective nurture and education and their socialization as valued and responsible contributing members of families and as citizens of society. These essential tasks, too, are often taken for granted but require considerable understanding and skill to ensure successful outcomes.

Recent research has documented a difference between *task accomplishment* and the role of *manager* in fulfilling many of these important family functions (Spitze, 1991; Thompson & Walker, 1991). Mederer (1993) found that " 'task' and 'management' allocation contribute independently and differently to perceptions of fairness and conflict about housework allocation" (p. 133). Barnett and Baruch (1988, p. 72) note that "responsibility" for or management of a set of tasks involves not just doing the tasks themselves but also "remembering, planning, and scheduling" to ensure task completion on an ongoing basis. Mederer (1993) and Barnett and Baruch (1988) also comment on the "invisibility" of these managerial roles for ensuring healthy family life. The role of manager in nonfamily organizational systems is often both highly valued and highly paid, whereas management aspects of the five family role areas just discussed—basic provision, leadership and decision making, household maintenance, dependents' care, and child rearing and socialization—are unpaid and often ignored. These issues will be examined in depth in Chapters 4 and 5.

Epstein and his colleagues (1982) note the importance of exploring in a family assessment such questions as "Does the person assigned a task or function have the power and skill necessary to carry it out? Is the assignment done clearly and explicitly? Can reassignment take place easily? Are tasks distributed and allocated to the satisfaction of family members?" They also observe that in healthy families, "All necessary family functions are fulfilled. Allocation is reasonable and does not overburden one or more members. Accountability is clear" (p. 125).

Beliefs and Rules

Another important area for understanding and exploration is the family's beliefs and rules; it is an arena that needs further empirical work. Beavers and his colleagues have identified "mythology" (i.e., family beliefs or worldview) as an important component in family assessment (Beavers, 1982; Lewis et al., 1976). They note that a holding in common or "congruence" among members' understanding of family life is critical. Satir (1988) has discussed the importance of explicit (rather than hidden or implicit) and appropriate system rules for healthy family life and noted the need for family rules to be updated and modified as the family develops and family members grow and change.

Satir (1988) emphasized the importance of rules about changing family rules, based on an open rather than closed set of basic family beliefs. Related to this understanding is Olson's concept of family "adaptability," defined as "the ability of a marital or family system to change its power structure, role relationships, and relationship rules in response to situational and developmental stress" (Olson & Lavee, 1989, p. 170; see also Olson et al., 1979; Thomas & Olson, 1993). Olson and his colleagues (1979) identify two healthy or balanced levels of adaptability, "structured" or "flexible," and two extreme or unhealthy levels, "chaotic" or "rigid."

Family rules are embedded in and flow from a broader family belief system (Blake, 1993) which, according to Bowen's (1978) model, results from the converging of belief systems brought from the partners' families of origin. In an article on parent-child relationships, Belsky (1990, p. 887) delineates a similar understanding with the use of Main, Kaplan, and Cassidy's (1985) term "internal working models." That is, a parent constructs relations with a child based on his or her own cognitive-affective representation, or "internal working model," which in turn is derived from experiences of and reflections on parent-child relationships from the parent's own childhood (Main & Goldwyn, 1984; see also Bowlby, 1969, 1988).

In early theoretical work, Boulding (1961) used the concept of *image*—that is, a person's image of the way the world operates—to understand behavior as guided by internal worldviews, or image systems. These images are not necessarily static, rigid, or unchangeable sets of beliefs. For most people, they are "internal working models," or fairly stable understandings of self and society which, based on new data and knowledge, can be updated, refined, and sometimes radically changed. Boulding (1961, p. 15) also discusses the concept of "universe of discourse" to describe the creation of *common* images or *shared* working models to guide the behaviors of two or more persons.

In summary, consensus has emerged on the importance of understanding a family system's "shared images," or beliefs held in common. For some troubled families, there may be no or few shared understandings, and family members may be in constant conflict over beliefs and rules derived from two or more very different individual family-of-origin internal working models to guide expectations and behaviors. When there are images held in common, these can include early hopes and visions that may or may not have been fulfilled in the marriage and current family life.

To elaborate, two partners (or a parent and other adults who share child-rearing roles and responsibilities) bring to family tasks learned images or internal working models of how a family "does and should" operate. These include beliefs, values, attitudes, rules for behavior, and so forth. One of the challenges faced in all family systems is to create shared images and understandings that are based on but often somewhat different from each of the imaginal worldviews of the individuals involved. The common images that explicitly or implicitly emerge over time out of ongoing interactions among family members form the base for stable patterns of behavior in the family system. These shared images can be elicited not only by identifying family rules and observing repetitious behavior sequences, including family rituals (Fiese, Hooker, Kotary, & Schwagler, 1993), but also by listening for family narratives, stories, and myths and making explicit the metaphors and analogies used by family members in discussions about their family (Hartman & Laird, 1987, p. 587).

This area of shared images is greatly in need of further empirical research and knowledge building. Many social work practitioners are aware of the deep satisfaction that comes from assisting a family in creating, or recreating, shared images of how "things will be done in this family." Practice experience makes clear that explicit and up-to-date rules and understandings regarding boundaries and affective involvement, roles and behaviors, and modes of communication can free families for successful problem solving, resulting in increased warmth, humor, and optimism (Beavers, 1982, p. 56).

Communication

For Olson and his colleagues, communication is one of the three key concepts (with cohesion and adaptability) in understanding family system functioning (Olson & Lavee, 1989; Thomas & Olson, 1993). The McMaster model defines communication as "the exchange of information within a family" (Epstein et al., 1982); for Satir (1988) this important aspect of family life has to do with "the ways people use to work out meaning with one another" (p. 4). Anderson and Carter (1990, p. 177) discuss the connection of communication with feelings and note that communication styles and patterns within the family "strongly influence the behavior" of family members.

Communication between family members may be verbal or nonverbal—facial expression, tone of voice, body posture and muscle tone, rate of breathing, gestures, and so forth (Satir, 1988). A practitioner who is able to "read" nonverbal communication in families can often observe a great deal about family functioning that family members may be unable or unwilling to verbalize, at least initially.

Olson and his colleagues identify six aspects of family communication for assessment: listening skills involving both empathy and attentive listening, speaker's skills encompassing both speaking for oneself and not speaking for others, self-disclosure, clarity, continuity in communication and the ability to track conversation, and an attitude of respect and regard (Thomas & Olson, 1993, p. 164). Both Satir (1988) and Epstein et al. (1982) emphasize the importance of clear, direct communication in which the verbal and nonverbal content of messages is "congruent" (Satir, 1988). Beavers (1982) discusses the importance of all family members speaking for themselves rather than making "mind-reading" statements for other members. Also significant is the development of effective negotiation skills that enable conflict resolution (rather than the family's getting stuck in unresolvable conflict).

It is through communication that families develop family system boundaries and cohesion, allocate tasks and manage organizational structures and roles, and share and agree on beliefs and rules for family life. Through effective communication, families solve problems and adapt to changes outside and inside the family system. Families and practitioners need to understand that ineffective communication patterns are learned behaviors and new skills for effective communication among all members of the family system can be learned and put into practice.

Family Life Cycles

A final critical aspect of a social systems approach to understanding and working with families is the concept of family life cycle. This provides a way of seeing family functioning and change developmentally. As summarized by Carter and McGoldrick (1988), families as social systems can be viewed as experiencing a series of socially normative stages: from two young adults becoming a couple (a two-person family), through stages of having and caring for an infant and having that infant grow into an adolescent, to the later stages of launching adult children, and in later life, experiencing the death of one's spouse and perhaps becoming dependent on children for frail-elder care. (See also Becvar & Becvar, 1993; McGoldrick, Heiman, & Carter, 1993.) It must be noted that this scheme simplifies, and perhaps at times oversimplifies, very complex processes; nonetheless, the life cycle model is useful for identifying family connections and change over time.

Carter and McGoldrick (1988) delineate six stages in the family life cycle: (a) single young adults, (b) new couples, (c) families with young children, (d) families with adolescents, (e) launching children and moving on, and (f) families in later life. Becvar and Becvar (1993, pp. 128-129) add three additional stages: "families with children" are subdivided into stages of "childbearing" and "families with a 'preschool-age child.'" In addition, "launching children and moving on" becomes the two stages of "launching center" and "middle-aged adults."

At the transition points for each of these stages, families face a number of issues and tasks, almost always involving the challenge of successfully negotiating morphogenetic or "second-order" changes (Carter & McGoldrick, 1988) in family boundaries, roles, beliefs, and rules. For example, the successful transition to being a couple includes developing boundaries, organizational structures, and shared images of family life. These images are based on and related to (but also different from) the systemic functioning of the families of origin of the two persons in the new committed relationship. Similarly, families experiencing the "launching children" transition face the challenge of (a) becoming a dyad once again, (b) enabling multiple exits and entrances (for example, young adults' leaving the family home and becoming financially and emotionally autonomous; involving adult children's spouses or partners in the family network; welcoming grandchildren into the family; deciding how and in what ways to include grandchildren's other grandparents in the family system; etc.), and (c) possibly negotiating care for elderly parents in the family of origin of each member of the couple and perhaps dealing with their death. Olson (1993) and Combrinck-Graham (1985) note that varying family patterns and styles are often needed, depending on the family life cycle stage. For example, in the first year of couplehood, "centripetal" experiences of closeness and connectedness may predominate, whereas families with adolescents may normally experience more "centrifugal" forces of distance and separateness.

Becvar and Becvar (1993) also include, in their complex view of family systems, the developmental life cycle stage of each person in the family as well as the "stages of a marriage" (p. 131). The life stage of each person is based on Erikson's view of psychosexual development. Four stages of marriage are delineated: honeymoon period (0-2 years), early marriage (2-10 years), middle marriage (10-25 years), and long-term marriage (25+ years). In their view, (a) the life stage and tasks of each person, (b) the developmental stage of the marriage, and (c) the life cycle stage of each of the couple's family of origin interact in a complex "dance" of growth, development, and change (see Becvar & Becvar, 1993, pp. 133-136).

Carter and McGoldrick (1988, p. 12) caution that such a normative view may ignore variation and change among persons and families. For example, for families who experience divorce, "dislocations of the family life cycle require additional steps to restabilize and proceed developmentally" (p. 22), and this stabilization has been found empirically to take at least 2 years. Similarly, remarriage families face developmental issues unique to this type of family system; the development of stable remarriage family patterns (boundaries and cohesion, organizational structures and roles, beliefs and rules, communication) may take "a minimum of two or three years" (p. 23). In addition, issues for nonmarital parents and for families without children are not addressed.

Further work is also needed with a focus on understanding developmental patterns based on diversity among cultures and societies (McGoldrick et al., 1993). In many parts of the world, young couples are expected to live, for at least a time, with one or the other of the couple's family of origin. In some cultures, the husband moves in with his new wife's family; in others, the wife comes to live with her husband's relatives. In some cultures, too, exits and entrances are more fluid, with children living, as needed, with a variety of relatives or others in the community. Examples include living in an extended-family network in some African American families or with tribal "kin" in some American Indian families.

In summary, an understanding of families as social systems, although it includes seeing each family member as an individual person, goes beyond that view to focus on relationships *between and among* family members *over time.* It includes attention to family boundaries and co-

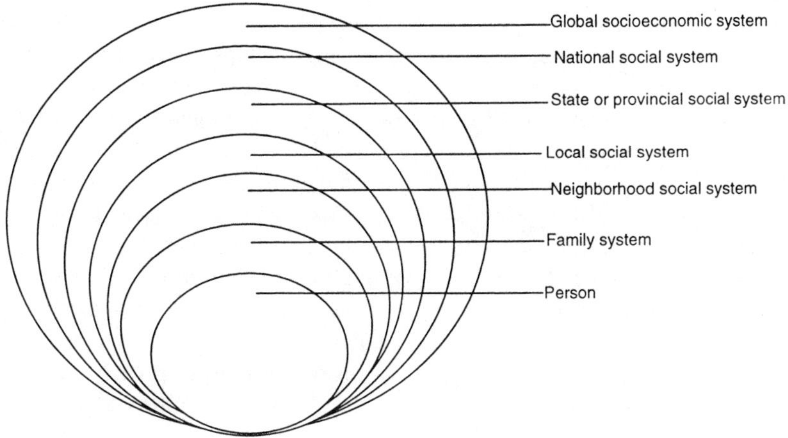

Figure 2.2. Multilevel Social Systems Model

SOURCE: Vosler and Ozawa (1992, p. 5). Copyright 1992 by Family Service America, Inc. Reprinted by permission of Families International, Inc.

hesion, organizational structures and roles, common beliefs and rules, communication, and life cycle stages. In addition, families, like family members, do not operate in a vacuum but develop and function in larger systems and structures.

LARGER SYSTEMS AND SOCIAL STRUCTURES

Just as families can be viewed as social systems that develop and function over time, Anderson and Carter (1990) discuss multiple social systems levels, including groups, communities, organizations, cultures, and society. Based on this understanding, Vosler and Nair (1993; see also Vosler & Ozawa, 1992) delineate seven nested social systems levels for understanding and possible assessment by social work and other human service professionals, shown in Figure 2.2: (a) the person, (b) the family system, (c) the neighborhood social system, (d) the local community social system, (e) the state or province as social system, (f) the national social system, and (g) the global social system.

This multilevel social systems model suggests that systems concepts from family studies can be applied to larger systems. Boundaries, roles and social structures, beliefs and rules, and communication flows are important in understanding how families are supported or negatively impacted by the system functioning of the larger systems in which families are embedded. In addition, this model suggests that at each level, structures and institutions are social constructions; that is, they evolve over time, and although change may be difficult, "second-order" change is possible, as what has been learned can be unlearned, and in place of old patterns, new patterns can become established.

The relationships between (a) persons and (b) the family system have been discussed above. Here, the five larger social systems levels— (c) neighborhood, (d) local community, (e) state, (f) nation, and (g) globe —are described briefly. A framework for analyzing each level is delineated, including a developmental view of social stability and social change.

The Neighborhood Social System

This level of larger systems can perhaps best be thought of as the "walking" community. Although some may argue that the automobile has eliminated geographical community in modern U.S. society, and although this may be true for suburban middle- and upper-middle-income families who have reliable transportation and drive easily to and from destinations (such as work, day care, schools, stores, services, recreation, etc.), for lower-income families, the presence or absence of services and social infrastructure in the "walking" neighborhood can be critical for family stability (see Graber, Haywood, & Vosler, in press; Vosler, 1989; Vosler & Ozawa, 1992).

In many inner-city U.S. neighborhoods abandoned by businesses and service agencies and blighted by poorly maintained housing owned by absentee landlords, families face overwhelming challenges in accessing goods and services that are essential to meet the basic needs of family members, including even food and shelter (see Wilson, 1987). In contrast, in high-rise housing estates in Singapore, planning has made possible the location of businesses (including food and retail shops), schools, community recreation facilities, and a variety of economic and social services (banks, repair shops, police, medical facilities, and elder services) in walking distance of low- and middle-income residential housing. In addition, all of these facilities employ local residents. (For a discussion and critique of Singapore's housing policies, see Blake, 1991.)

The Local Community Social System

The viability of neighborhoods often depends on the operation of economic and political organizational structures in a local community system, such as a town, city, or county. A critical initial question for analysis, particularly in large metropolitan areas, is how boundaries are drawn between the various public and private social institutions. Based on governmental structuring, part of a metropolitan area can have an adequate tax base for excellent schools and other social infrastructures, whereas adjacent neighborhoods may lack the resources for even minimally adequate police and fire protection, schools, and other services.

Such disjunctures do not bode well for the healthy functioning of the community as a whole, for it follows that families unable to meet basic needs will not have the means to raise healthy children and youth. The result is that some families over time become more and more of a burden for community-wide justice and social service structures. The challenge for political and economic leadership in the entire local community (city, county, town), with citizen participation based on shared beliefs and values, is to work to change old patterns that exclude particular groups and invest in social (and economic) infrastructures that support all families in healthy functioning.

The State as Social System

States as geographical and governmental social systems also have within their boundaries organizational patterns and structures that can be described, mapped, and analyzed. Economic institutions, both private and public, including tax systems, need to be examined. For example, financing and funding sources and levels for economic development, transportation, housing, income support, and social services for middle- and low-income families need to be analyzed. These include health care (e.g., Medicaid; school lunch programs; the Women, Infants, and Children [WIC] nutrition program), mental health and substance abuse treatment programs, education (e.g., Head Start, Parents as Teachers, disparities and possible subsidies in per-pupil funding across school districts), child care and after-school programming, youth recreation programs, and income supports (e.g., child support; Aid to Families With Dependent Children [AFDC]; tax exemptions for children, elderly dependents, child care; etc.).

In addition, political leadership and power, and citizen participation or exclusion, can be delineated. Cultural beliefs and values can be described. From a social systems perspective, such patterns can be understood as evolving social constructions in historical perspective and thus subject to second-order changes. Current changes in federal policies, especially in block grants to states for a variety of social welfare programs, are already forcing state legislators to rethink state-level funding patterns for programs and services. These changing patterns open up the possibility for both positive and negative changes at state, local, and neighborhood levels, with concomitant shifts (for better or worse) in supports for families and family members.

The Nation as Social System

Although extremely complex and often overwhelming, nations can be viewed as social systems, made up of smaller social systems (states, counties, and cities), with agreed on (or changing, as in the case of the Soviet Union and Russia) boundaries and organizational structures unique to this level of system functioning. In a recent book, Galbraith (1992) discusses the political economy of the United States in terms of belief systems ("the culture of contentment"), power structures, and resulting economic consequences for lower-income persons and families. In this analysis, he makes clear that national policies make a difference in social structures, and therefore in citizens' lives, throughout the social system that is the nation of the United States of America.

The current rethinking of federal versus state and local responsibilities has far-reaching implications for economic development and stabilization (e.g., farm subsidies, transportation systems), education, health care access (Medicare, Medicaid, national health care reform), income support (minimum wage levels, social security, AFDC, food stamps), and social services (housing and child care subsidies, child protective and child welfare services, youth and displaced worker education and training, etc.). Decision makers, including voters, need empirically based knowledge of benefits, costs, and long-term consequences for families of a variety of alternative policies and proposals for change.

The Global Social System

Although the global system is the most complex and least understood social system level, some social workers and others are beginning to see that Planet Earth is in fact a unitary ecological system that encompasses a variety of social and organizational structures (Hoff, 1992; Hoff & McNutt, 1994; Hoff & Polack, 1993; Rogge, 1993). It is also clear that

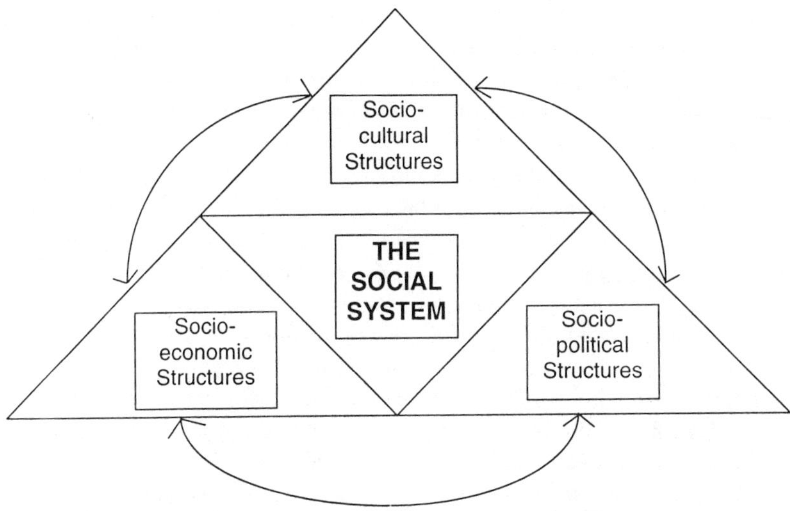

Figure 2.3. Components of Social Systems

social workers and other human service professionals cannot afford to ignore the emerging global socioeconomic system, for its operation affects not only Third World countries (Lewis, 1992) but also the viability of economic security and social welfare schemes in industrialized nations, including the United States.

Structures, Organizations, Agencies, and Policies

At each of these social systems levels, organizations, agencies, and policies can be described and discussed. A helpful framework for analyzing social systems—whether neighborhoods or nations—is shown in Figure 2.3, which is based on work done by participants of the Institute of Cultural Affairs (ICA, 1981). In this framework, a social system can be seen as made up of at least three sets of social structures, which interact to form the whole that is the particular social system. These social system components are (a) socioeconomic structures, (b) sociopolitical structures, and (c) sociocultural structures. These substructures can be seen as corresponding to some degree with the social science disciplines of economics, political science, and anthropology and sociology.

Economists have hitherto tended to describe and prescribe economic structures as if they were separate from the context of the larger social system. A social systems view suggests that social workers and other human service professionals collaborate with economists and others in understanding and assessing economic structures in relation to other components of the social system and in relation to consequences for all members constituting the particular social system under investigation.

Similarly, a particular set of political structures may support or hinder healthy functioning of social systems at various systems levels. Assessment of these structures by practitioners and researchers should include an understanding of who does and does not vote, who holds power to make decisions, how the social welfare system works and is supported, and how police and justice systems work in relation to participation and the functioning of the economic system.

Related to and affected by both socioeconomic and sociopolitical substructures are the sociocultural structures of any social system. These include shared cultural and religious belief systems, values, norms and rules, as well as the means through which these are conveyed to future generations (i.e., educational structures). According to this view, if there are clear and explicit values, beliefs, and rules held in common, these images will help to stabilize the operation of the political economy. Alternatively, where values and belief systems are implicit and not shared by most members of the social system, conflict in this set of structures is likely to spill over into conflict over economic and political structures, and vice versa.

A Developmental Social Construction View

The multilevel social systems model depicted in Figures 2.1 and 2.2 incorporates the view that social systems evolve and change—or can be changed—over time. No particular set of economic, political, and cultural substructures is set in stone as an immovable barrier to change. As in family systems, however, there may be powerful tendencies for the homeostasis of current organizational structures and patterns. On the other hand, particularly in times of social crisis, major morphogenetic changes—that is, structural changes in economic, political, and cultural patterns—may be possible at one or a number of system levels.

In summary, for competent professional work with families and their members, a clear understanding by practitioners and researchers of larger social systems and structures is necessary for effective assessment and intervention. Although it is clear that an individual practitioner may have expertise and time for work at only two or perhaps three system levels (for example, work with families and work through advocacy structures with and on behalf of families at the local and state level), a multilevel view of larger systems and structures widens the lens for understanding and assessment, particularly in work with families stressed by economic changes, unemployment, or poverty.

FAMILY STRESS AND COPING

The concept of *stress* has emerged in the biological and social sciences as a way of understanding linkages between various levels of system functioning. Stress has been viewed as the process by which demands in the social environment are translated into unhealthy responses by the person, both psychologically and physically (Baum, Davidson, Singer, & Street, 1987). Lazarus and Folkman (1984) define psychological stress as "a relationship between the person and the environment that is appraised by the person as taxing or exceeding his or her resources and endangering his or her well-being" (p. 21). Psychological stress can be associated with biochemical changes in the body, leading to physical symptoms, illness, and even death (Baum et al., 1987).

At the family system level, a family stress and coping model has been developed, based on work by Hill (1949, 1958) and further elaborated by McCubbin et al. (1980; McCubbin & Patterson, 1983). The components of the ABCX Model of Family Stress and Coping, shown in Figure 2.4, are (A) the *event,* (B) the family's *resources* for coping with the event, (C) the family's *definition* of (or beliefs about) the event. These three (A, B, C) combine to produce the *level of crisis* (X), which is defined as "the amount of incapacitatedness or disorganization in the family where resources are inadequate" (McCubbin et al., 1980, p. 127).

Potentially stressful events faced by families and their members can be normative (McCubbin & Figley, 1983) or catastrophic (Figley & McCubbin, 1983). *Normative* events are often associated with the growth and development of individual family members and with family life cycle transitions and changes. Each transition in the family life cycle—from single young adults to a married couple, from married couple to a family with young children, from a family with young children to a family with adolescents, from a family with adolescents to a family launching children and moving on, from a launching family to

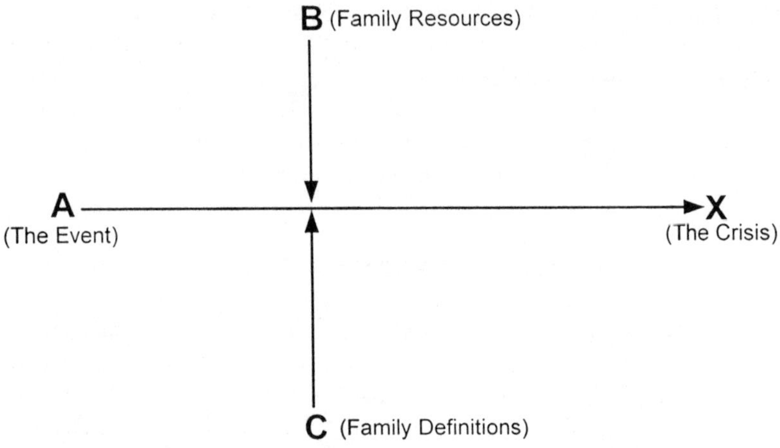

Figure 2.4. ABCX Model of Family Stress and Coping

a family in later life—may be experienced as stressful, depending on resources available to and within the family, and on the family's definitions of and beliefs about change, particularly *this* change.

If, for example, a newly married couple, despite both partners working full-time, is struggling financially to provide rent and food for themselves (B = limited resources), then an unplanned pregnancy and subsequent transition to being a family with an infant (A) may be a very difficult time of crisis (X) even though the couple may believe that this is an exciting and fulfilling change (C). In another family, in which resources (B) are adequate, but where loss and grief are difficult unresolved issues (C = family definitions and beliefs), the transition to the stage of being a family in later life (A) may be a time of especially high anxiety and distress (X).

At each transition point (A), there are likely to be changes in resource demands (B) as well as the necessity for changes in basic beliefs, rules, boundaries, roles, and organizational structures. These important changes will be guided by the family's shared definitions and images of this change event and of the process of change itself (C).

Other normative stressful events or situations for families identified and discussed by McCubbin and Figley (1983) include being a minority family (McAdoo, 1982), living in a rural area of the United States, being

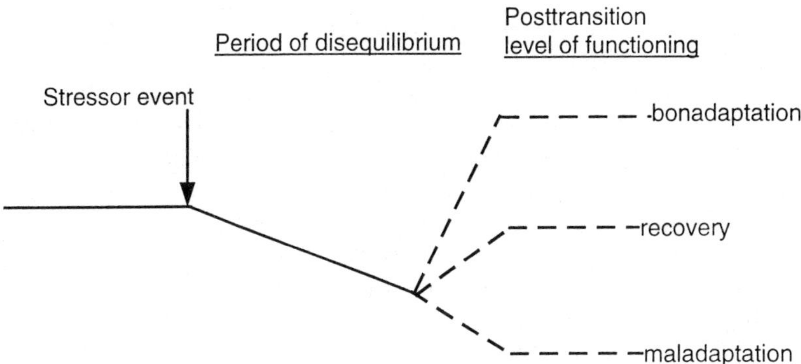

Figure 2.5. Family Transition Process Following a Stressor Event

a dual-career family (Skinner, 1982), decisions about balancing work and family, divorce, single parenting, adaptation to limited or decreased income, and stepparenting.

Nonnormative events or family *catastrophes* discussed by various authors (Figley & McCubbin, 1983) include natural disasters, illness (Rolland, 1993), drug abuse, abandonment, death, unemployment (Moen, 1982), rape, war, and captivity. Such events (A) may tax the coping ability of the family's shared understandings of life (C), overwhelm financial and emotional resources (B), and leave family members feeling out of control and exhausted (X) (McCubbin & Patterson, 1983).

In addition, researchers have documented the impact of *stress pileup* involving interaction between fairly common low-level stressors that together "add up" to a crisis (see, e.g., Vosler & Proctor, 1990). The tendency of stressors to build on one another over time has been called the Double ABCX Model (McCubbin & Patterson, 1983). The stress pileup concept is being used to explore the impact on families of chronic illness (McCubbin et al., 1982) and of chronic poverty.

Related to an understanding of family stress and coping *over time* is the "roller coaster course of adjustment" (McCubbin et al., 1980, p. 125) depicted in Figure 2.5. This involves an event followed by a period of disorganization and efforts to cope with the event, resulting in several potential levels of postcrisis adjustment, including (a) recovery to the former level of functioning (i.e., reestablishing of system homeostasis), (b) maladaptation (morphogenetic reorganization at a lower level of functioning), or (c) bonadaptation (morphogenetic reorganization at a higher level of functioning) (see McCubbin & Patterson, 1983; Mederer & Hill, 1983).

This view of systemic adaptation and change emphasizes that the transition period in a time of crisis is ambivalent in the same sense that the Chinese character for "crisis" includes the concepts of "danger" and "opportunity." The challenge of one or more stressful events in the life of a family presents family members with the opportunity, over time, to reconstruct their shared beliefs, roles, boundaries, and communication patterns and develop structures that lead to better adaptation and functioning.

In the remainder of this book, I focus on current knowledge for practice regarding the impact of larger systems on families in three interrelated arenas, based on family stress and coping theory integrated with the multilevel social systems model of larger systems and structures. In Chapter 4, I review research on the now fairly normative stress in families regarding balancing work in the labor force with "family work." Particular attention will be paid to dual-earner families in which both parents must be employed to provide adequately for the family's needs. Chapter 6 contains an overview of studies that have dealt with the "nonnormative," or catastrophic stress of unemployment of one (or both) provider(s) in the family. In Chapter 8, I review and discuss emerging understandings of the impact of stress pileup from poverty—particularly chronic poverty—on family members and family system functioning. Each of these arenas is highlighted here to delineate how they are related to a multilevel social systems—and developmental (over time) stress and coping—approach to understanding and working with families.

Work and Families

In the U.S. in the past two decades, many families with children have found it necessary for both parents to enter the labor force for the family to remain in the middle class (Menaghan & Parcel, 1991). Some women are employed full-time by choice and have—along with their husbands —careers with salaries sufficient to allow them to purchase household and child care services. In many families, both parents must work full-time to provide for basic needs, including food, shelter, personal items, health care, education, and recreation (Wilkie, 1991). For families in which two people work full-time to fulfill the provider role, other family and parental roles—including household management, care of elderly or disabled family members, and the raising of children—are often still left to the woman (Thompson & Walker, 1991). In some cases, tasks may be left undone with subsequent difficulties for all family members over how to manage frustration and role overloads.

Social science and professional knowledge building have too often focused primarily—or even exclusively—on the family system to try to "solve" this problem of role overload. Viewed from a larger perspective, the difficulty lies at least partially in the arrangements in contextual (neighborhood, local, state, and national) socioeconomic and political structures. In these structures, there has been a shift from higher-wage jobs with benefits that enable one person working full-time to fulfill the role of family provider to rising numbers of low-wage, often part-time jobs without benefits—forcing both parents to struggle to provide for the family (see, e.g., Wallace & Rothschild, 1988). The stress from role overload can, over time, potentially lead to escalating family conflict, marital disruption, and even family violence. Although the struggle to balance the roles entailed in employed work and family work is certainly a normative stress in today's society, solutions must be sought not only within the family system but at larger system levels as well. Detailed discussion of these issues can be found in Chapters 4 and 5.

Unemployment and Families

Although unemployment has in the past been viewed as a nonnormative, even catastrophic, event, many U.S. families today struggle to cope with this potentially devastating stressor (Voydanoff, 1991). Particularly in families in which both parents must work to make ends meet, the layoff of one of the providers can throw the family finances into a major crisis, with concomitant systemic reverberations including anxiety, depression, and family conflict (Vosler, 1994).

In local economies where large numbers of workers are laid off, reemployment may be difficult. Even when a job is found, there may be a substantial drop in wages resulting in the need to reconstruct family organizational structures, roles, and rules. In addition, where reemployment is unstable and unemployment occurs again, the family may begin to slide toward poverty and experience vulnerability to other stressful events, such as relocation resulting in the loss of supportive networks of family and friends, stress-related illnesses, and the increasing likelihood that parents will have to settle for part-time unstable employment without benefits (McLeod & Kessler, 1990).

The stress pileup from repeatedly reorganizing family life based on changing parental employment and shifting family finances and housing can lead to maladaptive family patterns. Such patterns can include chronic conflict or violence, family dissolution and cutoffs, hopelessness, drug abuse, and untreated stress-related physical or mental illnesses in family members. Family social work practice that focuses only on individual family members or even the family system will not resolve the need for stable employment with benefits and at wages that provide adequate access to basic necessities for all family members. An understanding of stress from the socioeconomic structuring of larger systems is needed, and multilevel interventions to change systems and structures is critical. These issues are further examined in Chapters 6 and 7.

Poverty and Families

Stress pileup in the family system can result, as well, from chronic poverty; and increasing numbers of families with children in the United States are experiencing this potentially disruptive stressor (Ellwood, 1988). Families with income below the poverty line—or even near the poverty line—in many cases are not able to afford, for example, both rent and utilities; or, if both are paid for the month, there may not be enough resources left to buy adequate food. Often, there is constant juggling of partial payments between such basic necessities as food, rent, utilities, medicine, school supplies, and children's shoes or a winter coat. Partial payments on rent can result, several months later, in a forced move or an eviction onto the street. Parents and children may then move in with extended family, at least temporarily, resulting in the need to restructure an expanded household system to accommodate additional members. When these sequences of events repeat at frequent intervals, family patterns are subject to constant, chaotic change, often resulting in maladaptive structures and behaviors. With repetition, a family homeostasis of sorts may evolve, based on the struggle to survive (Hollingshead & Redlich, 1958) and leading to family beliefs that focus on the here and now—because, in the family's experience, futuristic planning seems useless and therefore not worth the energy.

For individuals growing up in such a system, particularly when there is accompanying chronic conflict, drug or alcohol abuse, or violence, the chaotic conditions may engender low self-esteem and a sense of personal ineffectiveness and hopelessness (Mirowsky & Ross, 1989). Without a different set of experiences in alternative social systems, young adults beginning families of their own can have difficulties envisioning stable, supportive, and nurturing family system patterns and can reconstruct in their new family the only kinds of structures they have known.

For some of these persons and families, positive change will be very slow, because the current family homeostasis may be experienced as the "only best way to survive." Stable changes in larger systems and structures may be necessary, including consistent access to affordable basic necessities, before the smaller component systems of persons and families can stabilize and new, more healthy patterns can be learned. Stable family system restructuring following a divorce or remarriage has been found to take at least 2 years, even when basic economic needs are met (Carter & McGoldrick, 1988). Whether this minimum time frame applies to other kinds of family restructuring processes needs further empirical investigation.

Certainly, not all families who encounter poverty experience concomitant destructive stress pileup (Lewis & Looney, 1983). It is clear, however, that the stable meeting of basic needs for all family members is a "necessary, albeit not sufficient, condition" for healthy family system functioning (Schneewind, 1989, p. 217). Further exploration of stress pileup as a result of chronic poverty and directions for multilevel systems knowledge building and practice are discussed in Chapters 8 and 9.

FAMILY DIVERSITY AND STRESS

An area that social work researchers and practitioners must take into account in using theory and research from a family systems perspective is family diversity. Knowledge building regarding families illustrates that different kinds of families experience different types of resources and stressors and may respond with differing belief systems, rules, roles, and organizational structures. These in turn influence the stressors families experience as well as families' access to coping resources. After a discussion of (a) the terms *normal* and *healthy* in relation to family systems, I delineate several types of differences in families, including (b) structural diversity, (c) ethnic variability, (d) stresses experienced by gay and lesbian families, (e) families with elderly or disabled members, and (f) families with large numbers of children.

Normal, Healthy Families

Defining normal or healthy families, like defining the term family itself, is critically important, as concept definitions frame both knowledge building and practice. Walsh (1982) sets forth four categories for discussion of family normality: (a) "asymptomatic family functioning," that is, "there are no recent symptoms of dysfunction or psychopathology in any family member"; (b) "optimal family functioning," that is, the family's functioning is compared with a set of "positive or ideal characteristics" for "healthy" families; (c) "average family functioning," that is, the family "fits a pattern that is typical or prevalent in most families"; and (d) "transactional family processes," an approach in which a variety of processes for family system "integration, maintenance, and growth" can be viewed as "normal," depending on the "temporal and social contexts" (pp. 5-6; see also Walsh, 1993).

As Walsh (1982, pp. 26-27) points out, a particular intervention model's "view of normal family functioning" is critical in understanding family "symptoms" and "goals of therapy." For example, according to the structural model of family therapy, normality or health in family systems is related to "boundaries [being] clear and firm" and there being a "hierarchy with [a] strong parental sub-system"; thus, interventions focus on attempts to "shift members' relative positions to disrupt malfunctioning pattern[s] and strengthen [the] parental hierarchy," and to "create clear, flexible boundaries" (Walsh, 1982, p. 26). For Satir, in healthy families, "self-worth [is] high," "communication [is] clear, specific, [and] honest," and "family rules [are] flexible, human, [and] appropriate"; therefore, interventions focus on fostering "direct, clear communication" and "individual and family growth through immediate shared experience" (Walsh, 1982, p. 27).

It must be noted that such models of family therapy have been criticized for "assuming" a two-parent, nuclear, often white middle-class U.S. family. (For extensive discussion of this issue, see Staples & Mirande, 1980.) Similarly, clinical research models and evaluation instruments have been criticized for early validation efforts that focused primarily on white middle-class U.S. populations, such as Olson's Circumplex Model (Olson et al., 1983), the Beavers-Timberlawn Family Evaluation Scale (Lewis et al., 1976), the McMaster Model of Family Functioning (Epstein et al., 1982), and the Moos Family Environment Scale (Moos & Moos, 1986). Moreover, some early studies of families tended inappropriately to generalize findings from white middle-class U.S. families to all families (Staples & Mirande, 1980).

Increasingly, researchers and practitioners are moving away from a "deficit model" or "cultural deviant approach" (Staples & Mirande, 1980, p. 159) for diverse family forms and paying attention to particular strengths and vulnerabilities of various types of families, in the context of structural arrangements within larger social systems. It is clear that society does, and must, value and encourage certain kinds of behaviors and arrangements for families, and discourage and even prohibit other behaviors. Behaviors to be prohibited include abuse and violence; sexual abuse; neglect; prejudice and discrimination, including racism and sexism; and other forms of exclusion based on sexual orientation, disability, age, and so forth. Definitions of normality and health in family systems must be continually evaluated, based on up-to-date empirical research and feedback from client families.

Structural Diversity

With increasing diversity among families in the United States, including rising numbers of single-parent and remarried families and intergenerational households, concern for impacts of these "nontraditional" structural arrangements on family functioning and on family members has intensified. Empirical studies of the past two decades have established that children can grow up healthy in a variety of family types (Ganong & Coleman, 1987; Ihinger-Tallman, 1986). This leads to the conclusion that negative stereotypes of single-parent and remarried households as "deficient" or "deviant"—stereotypes based on the nuclear family as the supposed "ideal norm"—must be set aside.

On the other hand, it is increasingly clear that given organizational structures in larger social systems, different kinds of families face varying stressors, with differing resources for coping. For example, in nuclear families in which both parents must work full-time to meet basic family needs, there is a vulnerability to role overload from family work roles, as well as to financial crisis should one or both parents experience unemployment. Single-parent households are extremely vulnerable to role overload because one parent is carrying two full-time jobs (employed work and family work). Because full-time employment may not provide enough income to meet basic needs, mother-only families are especially vulnerable to poverty and a host of additional stressors that accompany chronic economic deprivation (Garfinkel & McLanahan, 1986; McLanahan & Booth, 1991). These include changes in residence, changes in employment, changes in child care arrangements and schools, lack of social supports, and resulting psychological distress.

Although remarriage may "solve" the "problem" of needing two parents in the labor force, the complexity of a remarried family can bring stress from internal family issues, such as parent-child conflicts and difficulties of stepparent and extended-family relationships (Hetherington, Stanley-Hagan, & Anderson, 1989; Vosler & Proctor, 1991). Particularly in remarriage families involving stepchildren, the new family system must reconstruct shared understandings and rules among all family members, rearrange roles and organizational structures, and work out boundaries for involvement of noncustodial parents in decision making about their biological children.

Similarly, intergenerational households often provide needed financial and social support among family members stressed by multiple roles or poverty. Like remarriage families, however, intergenerational family systems must deal with the complexity of constructing, among multiple family members, shared understandings about boundaries, roles, family decision making, and rules for discipline and behavior.

In each of these structurally diverse kinds of families (nuclear, extended, single-parent, and remarried households), there is a great deal of variability, based on multiple internal and external system factors (e.g., socioeconomic status, organizational structures, family history, etc.). Continuing empirical work is needed to understand stress and healthy patterns for coping in a variety of family structural forms.

Ethnic Variability

In an increasingly multiethnic, multicultural U.S. society, researchers and practitioners have begun to pay increasing attention to ethnic and racial diversity among U.S. families (Proctor et al., 1995). In their 1980 decade review of the literature on minority families, Staples and Mirande (1980) discussed the research biases deriving from a "cultural deviant" approach to families whose ethnic background is Asian, African American, Hispanic, or Native American. Such families have been subjected to negative stereotypes, and researchers have assumed that "different" meant "deficient." Alternatively, the "cultural variant" approach depicts a variety of family social system arrangements as "different, but functional, family forms" (Staples & Mirande, 1980, p. 159).

A developmental social systems stress and coping view of families enables practitioners as well as family members to understand current functioning in the context of both family and ethnic history. Different ethnic groups have had very different experiences over the past decades within U.S. state and national social systems (Hill, 1993; Marger, 1991). These include the decimation of sovereign Native American nations and domination of African Americans through slavery and segregation. Individuals and families in particular ethnic groupings may have had divergent experiences leading to heterogeneous family beliefs and structures (Davis & Proctor, 1989). Researchers and practitioners must pay attention to strengths and vulnerabilities for a variety of families.

The emphasis in some recent research on family strengths and "resiliency" (Chadiha, 1992) is an important emerging theme. Such characteristics as "family unity," kinship and other "interfamily cooperation," "role flexibility," and the "ability to mobilize . . . resources" (Chadiha, 1992, p. 544) from such social networks as extended-family, religious, neighborhood, ethnic, or tribal communities have been identified as salient in resilient families. Understanding and building on these strengths is a key aspect of professional practice (Hopps, Pinderhughes, & Shankar, 1995). Waldegrave (1990) recommends "cultural partnerships" and the use of a "cultural consultant" in cross-cultural work with families, noting that a practitioner from "the same culture as the client's will more easily understand the significance given in a story . . . [and] will also be more informed about possible new meanings . . . , drawing significantly on the culture" (p. 33). Proctor et al. (1995) note the importance of increasing the number of nonwhite professionals to work with their respective family groupings.

The impact of stress from racial prejudice and discrimination, economic disadvantage, and poverty must also be taken into account in understanding the functioning of many ethnic minority families. African American men in particular are increasingly economically disadvantaged, facing high unemployment, unstable employment, low earnings, and poverty (Chadiha, 1992; Hill, 1993; Wilson, 1987; for Hispanic families, see Vega, 1991). Experiences of unstable employment and poverty have been shown to have destabilizing effects on both family formation (Chadiha, 1992; Wilson, 1987) and family system maintenance (McLoyd, 1990; Taylor, Chatters, Tucker, & Lewis, 1991; Vega, 1991). In work with and knowledge building for understanding families from a variety of ethnic backgrounds, attention to beliefs and structures at multiple system levels within and outside the family is critical. Strengths must be identified and enhanced. Where larger contextual systems and structures do not provide needed opportunities and resources, or are actively detrimental to healthy family functioning (such as promoting negative stereotypes of particular variant family forms or cultural styles), interventions at multiple levels must be planned and implemented with and on behalf of families and family members.

Gay and Lesbian Families

Like many minority families, households with one or more gay or lesbian members often face negative stereotypes and social stigma (Laird, 1993). In addition, depending on local and state-level system structures, lesbian and gay parents may encounter difficult legal issues in such areas as child custody, parental rights, and foster care and adoption. They may also face home ownership restrictions and lack of access to a partner's employee family benefits, such as health care, child care, and social security and other retirement provisions (Green & Bozett, 1991).

Although myths and fears abound regarding children raised by gay or lesbian parents, and the empirical research base is somewhat limited and needs to be expanded, Green and Bozett (1991) conclude, after a careful literature review, that "children . . . who have lesbian or gay parents are comparable to the children of heterosexual parents. Their parents' sexual orientation is not the determining factor in their health and well-being" (p. 206). Their review includes children of gay fathers and children of lesbian mothers and addresses various aspects of children's functioning, including gender role behaviors, peer relationships, separation and individuation, and self-esteem.

Among gay and lesbian families, there is wide structural variability, including heterosexually married gay and lesbian parents, gay and lesbian stepparent families, and adoptive and foster parenting arrangements (Bozett, 1987). Because of advances in medical technology, an emerging option for gay and lesbian couples is parenthood through alternative fertilization or artificial insemination (Pies, 1987). Pies (1987, p. 165) notes that this practice highlights a number of social, psychological, and ethical issues for both families and society.

Miller (1987, p. 178) notes that professional practice with gay and lesbian persons can involve work with a number of "complicated family dynamics." Bozett (1987, p. 235) recommends a gay/lesbian specialty in family social science to develop better understandings of strengths and stressors in these families.

Families With Elderly or Disabled Members

Because of the rising need for multiple providers for families with dependents to meet basic needs (Wilkie, 1991), families with a disabled or poor elderly member are at risk for stress from both poverty and role overload. Disability of one of the parental providers can decimate the family's financial base. As Ellwood (1988) points out, "Virtually no governmental programs offer protection for people who suffer a short-term injury or disability that was not sustained on the job" (p. 95), and low-income parents are unlikely to be able to afford substantial private disability insurance.

Although poverty among the elderly has been declining overall (Ozawa, 1991), inflation over the past decades has negatively and disproportionately affected retired and disabled persons (Aldous, Ganey, Trees, & Marsh, 1991), making low-income individuals in these groups more vulnerable to financial distress. Families of these persons can subsequently experience social pressures to provide financial and other types of support. Although this may be appropriate when there are sufficient resources to make this possible, in families already stressed by multiple provider and family work roles, additional financial and emotional stress may tip the balance in the family into strained relationships and escalating conflict (Brubaker, 1991; Mancini & Blieszner, 1991).

Large Families

In the urban-industrial U.S. national social system, children are now "liabilities" rather than "assets" (Huber, 1988; Ozawa, 1989). Like disabled or elderly persons in the family, they are more likely to be low-income- or no-income-producing "economic units" in the household. Consequently, families with larger numbers of dependent children increase their likelihood of stress from role overload, as well as from vulnerability to unemployment or family system instability from chronic poverty.

When working with low-income families, practitioners must be aware that the 1995 national poverty guidelines (U.S. Department of Health and Human Services [U.S. DHHS], 1995) indicate that the absolute minimum *net* annual income required to meet basic survival needs for families with two parents and two dependent children (i.e., a four-member family unit), is $15,150; a family with two parents and six children (i.e., an eight-member family unit) must have at least $10,240 *more*—or $25,390. One parent working full-time full-year at minimum wage ($4.25 per hour, 40 hours per week, 52 weeks in a year) will gross (before taxes and any expenses) only $8,840; two parents working full-time full-year at this rate will gross only $17,680. (Note that these gross income figures do not take into account child care costs, which for one child for out-of-home care can be "from $1,500 to $10,000 per year, with the majority of parents paying $3,000 per year for child care services"; Friedman, 1986, pp. 80-81). Ozawa and Wang (1993) note that expecting minimum-wage parents to work their way off government welfare programs and out of poverty is a very unrealistic national social system goal.

It must be emphasized that not all large families are poor, nor do a majority of poor families have large numbers of children. In the current uncertain employment environment of the U.S. national social system, however, many larger families with dependent children do face greater vulnerability to stress from economic hardship and poverty, particularly when one or more of the provider parents faces unemployment from layoffs, plant closings, or other structural economic shifts in larger social systems.

SUMMARY

A social systems approach to family practice must (a) clearly define the concept of family, and (b) integrate multiple systems levels (person, family, neighborhood, local community, state, nation, and globe) with social construction, developmental (including family life cycle), and stress and coping theoretical perspectives to address diverse families and family issues. Woven throughout must be (c) an understanding of different kinds of households, including sources of internal and external stress for a variety of U.S. families in a complex multicultural society.

Building on this multilevel social systems model, Chapter 3 provides an overview of specific practice tools and methods for systemic work with families.

Chapter 3

FAMILY SYSTEMS IN CONTEXT
Applications and Tools for Practice

Focusing primarily on tools for understanding and working for changes *within* the *family* social system, this chapter provides an overview of practice tools and methods for systemic work with families. Chapters 5, 7, and 9 more specifically describe methods and tools for work with families in which changes at *larger* social systems levels are necessary for social work practice to be effective.

In this chapter, I first address some unique features of systemic family practice. Next, specific tools for work with families as social systems are delineated. Because systemic practice focuses on relationships between two or more family members as well as relationships outside the family, the importance of engaging multiple family members is discussed. With increased professional awareness of the importance of understanding family diversity, the practice strategy of team consultation is outlined. Models and methods for systemic intervention and evaluation are described. Finally, I discuss implications for multilevel social systems knowledge building and change.

THINKING SYSTEMICALLY

Systemic work with families does not eliminate attention to specific family members and their individual needs. The unique character of work with families as social systems, however, is that the added dimensions of relationships between family members and between the family and larger social systems become integral components of assessment and intervention processes. Beliefs and shared working models in the current sociocultural subsystem of U.S. society today tend to focus on the individual—often to the exclusion of social systems of any kind, including families, communities, and larger social structures (Bellah, Madsen, Sullivan, Swidler, & Tipton, 1985). As a result of this limiting individualistic view of human behavior—and a concomitant and sometimes exclusive professional focus on individual problems and "treatment" therapies—work with clients whose difficulties are embedded in stress from family functioning or structural inadequacies in larger systems can be ineffective; the larger issues need to be acknowledged and addressed.

The multilevel social systems model provides a wider lens for social workers and other human service professionals to see all—or more—of the pieces in the lives of families, and therefore to assess, understand, and work with families more comprehensively and holistically. The distinct way of thinking (i.e., "common working model") provided by this multilevel model requires tools for assessment and intervention as well as evaluation models and processes that enable practitioners and family members to *see* and then *decide* about participating in change efforts at one *or more* systems levels.

The theoretical perspective delineated in the model incorporates developmental social science knowledge building as a key process in social work practice. Empirical assessment of families in the context of larger social systems as well as evaluation of interventions and change efforts become essential components of professional practice, not only to provide accountability but also to contribute to ongoing professional knowledge building. The relationship between assessment and evaluation and the development of valid and reliable common measures for ongoing research, theory development, and knowledge building are critical areas for continuing work by social work practitioners and researchers.

TOOLS FOR FAMILY ASSESSMENT

A number of important tools for internal assessment of the family as a social system have been developed both within the family therapy movement and by social workers and other human service professionals. (For overviews of the development of family therapy, see Becvar &

Becvar, 1993; Kolevzon & Green, 1985.) The following specific tools for assessment and work with families in the context of larger social systems are discussed: (a) the multigenerational genogram; (b) the household ecomap, including relationships with extended family, friends, social and religious institutions, community groups, and other support networks; (c) family mapping of roles, including, for example, daily or weekly time and task routines; (d) family income, expenditures, and assets; (e) family beliefs, rules, rituals, and narratives, including ethnic, religious, and cultural practices and family sculpting; (f) family communication patterns; (g) the family life chronology and time line, including family life cycle transitions; (h) the home visit, including a neighborhood walk; (i) overview of larger social systems and knowledge of policies and programs at local, state, national, and global levels; and (j) some current measures for assessing overall internal family as well as individual family members' functioning.

The Multigenerational Genogram

An early tool developed for visualizing and understanding systemic family relationships is the family genogram (for a detailed discussion of its use in family assessments, see McGoldrick & Gerson, 1985). Using symbols (see Figure 3.1) for individual family members (circles for females; squares for males) and generational and other relationship lines and symbols to delineate births, marriages, separations, divorces, adoptions, miscarriages, deaths, twins and other sibling relationships, household boundaries, family cutoffs, illnesses (including mental illnesses), key dates in the family history, and so forth, a readable "picture" can be painted of complex multigenerational family realities and patterns (Figure 3.2).

As Mattaini (1993) points out, this visualization is worth a thousand words for both practitioners and family members in understanding family strengths as well as internal family stresses, anxiety, and pain. In developing the genogram, the social worker—or professional team—and family members together delineate the complexity of the family system (for example, remarriage relationships), boundaries, and current cutoffs within and across generations as well as sources of family cohesion, fragmentation, or rigidity. Although the genogram is not designed to provide specific guidelines for interventions, it does assist with an overall assessment for understanding the multigenerational context of current family system functioning.

A. Symbols to describe basic family membership and structure (include on genogram significant others who lived with or cared for family members—place them on the right side of the genogram with a notation about who they are).

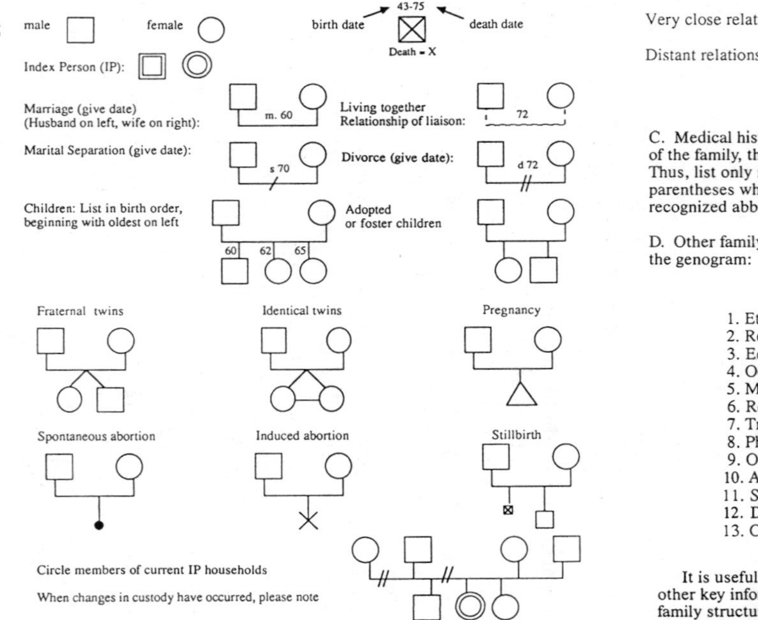

B. Family interaction patterns. The following symbols are optional. The clinician may prefer to note them on a separate sheet. They are among the least precise information on the genogram, but may be key indicators of relationship patterns the clincian wants to remember:

Very close relationship

Conflictual relationship

Distant relationship

Estrangement or cutoff (give dates if possible):

Fused and conflictual

C. Medical history. Since the genogram is meant to be an orienting map of the family, there is room to indicate only the most important factors. Thus, list only major or chronic illnesses and problems. Include dates in parentheses where feasible or applicable. Use DSM-III categories or recognized abbreviations where available (e.g., cancer CA; stroke CVA).

D. Other family information of special importance may also be noted on the genogram:

1. Ethnic background and migration date
2. Religion or religious change
3. Education
4. Occupation or unemployment
5. Military service
6. Retirement
7. Trouble with law
8. Physical abuse or incest
9. Obesity
10. Alcohol or drug abuse (symbol = ◪ ◯)
11. Smoking
12. Dates family members left home: LH '74
13. Current location of family members

It is useful to have a space at the bottom of the genogram for notes on other key information: This would include critical events, changed in the family structure since the genogram was made, hypotheses, and other notations of major family issues or changes. These notations should always be dated, and should be kept to a minimum, since every extra piece of information on a genogram complicates it and therefore diminishes its readability.

Figure 3.1. Symbols Used in Genograms

SOURCE: *The Changing Family Life Cycle*, 2nd ed. by Carter and McGoldrick (1988). Copyright 1988 by Allyn and Bacon. Reprinted by permission.

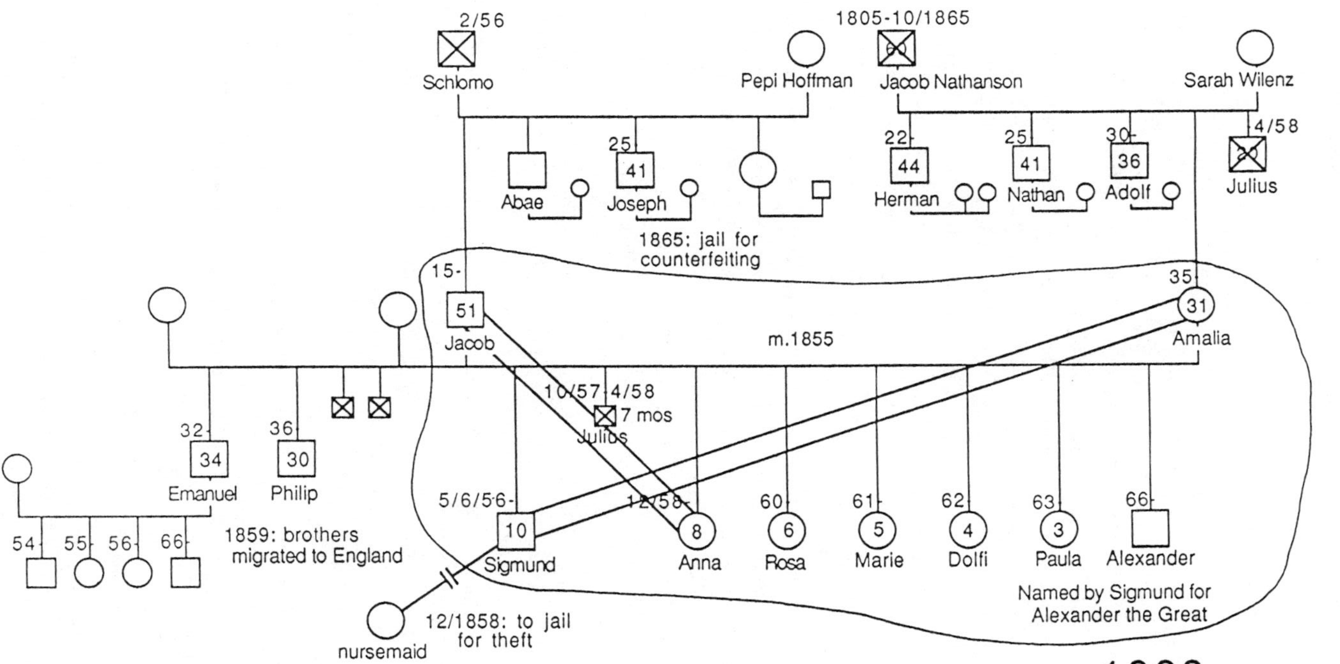

Figure 3.2. A Multigenerational Genogram

SOURCE: *The Changing Family Life Cycle*, 2nd ed. by Carter and McGoldrick (1988). Copyright 1988 by Allyn and Bacon. Reprinted by permission.

The Household Ecomap

The ecomap, a tool for professional assessment and work with families, is used less frequently than the genogram but is often more important for effective social work practice with families under stress from larger social systems. It was developed by Meyer (1976, 1983) and Hartman and Laird (1983; see also Mattaini, 1993).

Using the ecomap, as shown in Figures 3.3 and 3.4, the social worker and family members can together identify sources of stress and support for individuals as well as the family as a whole. The ecomap is usually based on the current residential household. In complex families—such as remarriage or extended families in which noncustodial children or other relatives may visit for periods of time—several ecomaps (or very complex ecomaps) may be developed to illuminate related sources of support and stress.

Development and discussion of the ecomap illustrate organizational structures and roles in the household as well as stresses from larger social systems. For example, in households where both parents are employed full-time outside the home, stress from role overload can result in conflict between partners, and frustration and even depression or other illness for one or more family members. On the other hand, if extended-family members are able to provide child care or other nonparental child care arrangements are stable and affordable, full-time employment for both parents may be a necessary, preferred, and satisfying arrangement for the family.

As the ecomap is being developed, relationships with extended family and friends can be explored, support from or frustration with community groups (e.g., church, synagogue, mosque, etc.) discussed, and access to benefits and services from institutions and other social agencies delineated. Examples include stable employment, schools and education programs, child care and youth programs, medical care, and social services. The ecomap is a tool for discerning the family's context for assessing both stressful relationships and supportive social networks, especially in the neighborhood and local social systems in which the current household is embedded.

Intrafamily Mapping

The family map focuses specifically on organizational structures, roles, and power *within* the current family household. It uses symbols to highlight partner and parent-child power relationships, boundaries,

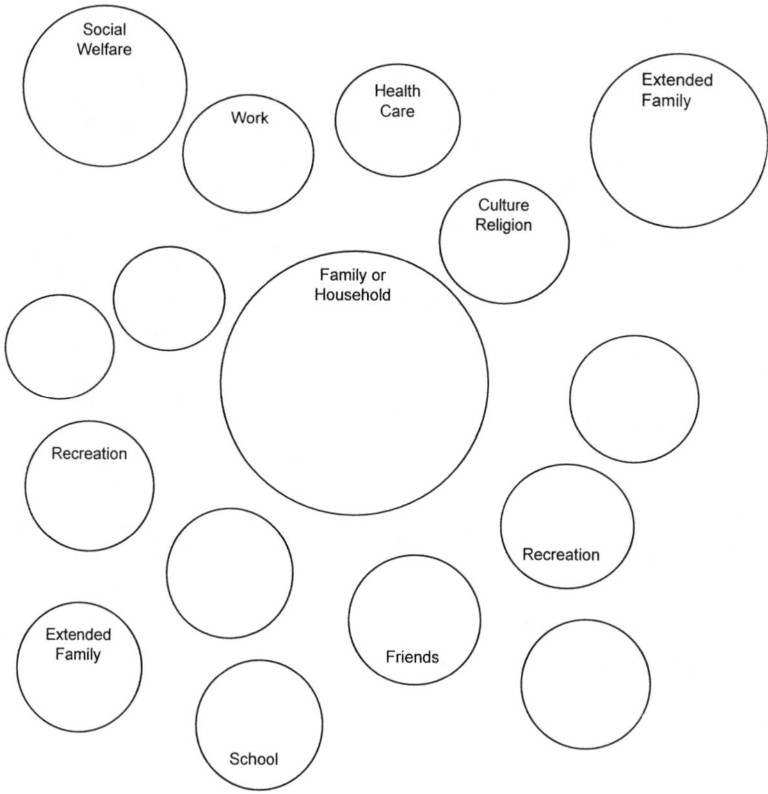

Figure 3.3. The Ecomap

SOURCE: Hartman (1978). Reprinted from Ann Hartman, *Social Casework,* October 1978. Used by permission of publisher, Families International, Inc.

NOTES: Fill in connections where they exist.

Indicate nature of connection with a descriptive word or by drawing different kinds of lines:

---------- for strong, - - - - - - for tenuous, -l-l-l-l-l for stressful.

Draw arrows along lines to signify flow of energy, resources, etc.: → → → → →.

Identify significant people and fill in empty circles as needed.

and conflicts (Mattaini, 1993; Minuchin, 1974). For example, family maps can be developed by the social worker and family members to identify clear or conflicted dyadic and triadic relationships, such as coalitions and detouring of conflict to a third family member (e.g., a child being triangulated into parents' marital conflict). Maps can also

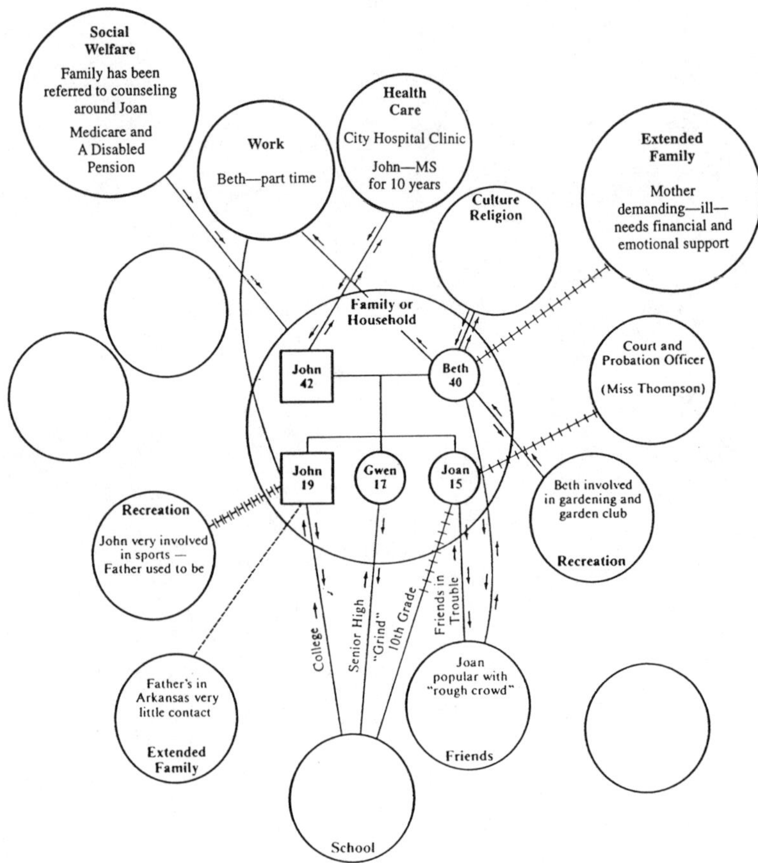

Figure 3.4. Ecomap of a Specific Household

SOURCE: Hartman (1978). Reprinted from Ann Harman, *Social Casework,* October 1978. Used by permission of publisher, Families International, Inc.

NOTES: Fill in connections where they exist.

Indicate nature of connection with a descriptive word or by drawing different kinds of lines: ---------- for strong, - - - - - - for tenuous, -l-l-l-l-l for stressful.

Draw arrows along lines to signify flow of energy, resources, etc.: → → → → →.

Identify significant people and fill in empty circles as needed.

be used to set goals for the future (e.g., shifting the focus of interventions from the child's behavior to the marital conflict) and to track and assess changes (e.g., reestablishing a marital alliance).

Discussion of the family map can help the practitioner and the family to identify who are the manager(s) and tasks helper(s) in family roles. These include earner(s)/provider(s), family leadership and decision making, household maintenance, dependents' care, and socialization of children and youth. Conflicts regarding role allocations (e.g., who does which tasks; the necessary time, energy, and commitment for task accomplishment; and how the manager role is fulfilled) for the parent(s) and other family members is mapped. Alignments, coalitions, and boundaries between and among partners and children should be mapped and assessed, leading to setting goals with the family for system changes.

Family Economy and Finances

As will be discussed in detail in subsequent chapters, household finances, including income, expenditures, and assets, are often a critical arena for exploration and assessment with families. Initially, a simple examination of monthly income and expenses (Figure 3.5) may reveal that this is a stable, functional component of family life. Alternatively, an initial discussion may signal that this is a primary source of stress and ongoing conflict in the family system.

Even for families in which income adequately covers normal expenses there may be dissatisfaction with current arrangements, roles, and expenditure patterns. Furthermore, family life cycle changes—an adolescent wanting a car, or uncertainty around changes in financial responsibility for an elderly parent—or sudden new or unexpected expenditures, such as medical care not covered by insurance, a move, a house fire, a burglary, or a car accident, may result in anxiety and conflict over current household economic arrangements.

For families in which there are income-expense deficits, assessment must examine the sources of financial difficulties. Are they related to family work role arrangements, poor money management, recent unemployment, employment instability, or long-term poverty? Exploration for understanding as well as for interventions and change must go beyond exclusive focus on the family system to an examination of neighborhood, local, state, and even national economic and social policies, programs, and structures.

Family Beliefs and Rules

Over time, families develop "internal working models," including sets of beliefs and rules for behavior that guide life in the family as a

MONTHLY HOUSEHOLD INCOME & EXPENDITURE				
	MY INCOME	ESTIMATED INCOME OF OTHER MEMBERS OF MY FAMILY	MONTHLY HOUSEHOLD EXPENDITURE	
NET/GROSS SALARY	______	______	HDB	______
ALLOWANCE/OVERTIME/ PENSION	______	______	PUB	______
			SC/CC	______
CHILD SUPPORT	______	______	MARKETING	______
CONTRIBUTIONS OUTSIDE THE HOUSEHOLD:			GROCERIES	______
A. FINANCIAL	______	______	TELEPHONE	______
B. FOOD	______	______	TRANSPORTATION:	
P.A.	______	______	1. OWN	______
REF NO. ______			2. FAMILY	______
APPROVAL DATE ______			EDUCATION:	
DURATION ______			1. SCHOOL FEES	______
RUAS:			2. ALLOWANCES	______
A. RENT	______	______	MEDICAL	______
B. UTILITIES	______	______	MISCELLANEOUS	______
REF NO. ______			OTHER (SPECIFY):	______
APPROVAL DATE ______			______	______
DURATION ______			______	______
			______	______
TOTAL	______	______		______
BALANCE I - E=	______	______		______

Figure 3.5. Monthly Household Income and Expenses

SOURCE: Research Casework Intake Form, Ang Mokio Family Service Centres, Singapore.

whole and that of individuals in the family. These working models pattern interactions, and influence not only the behaviors but also the cognitions and emotions of family members.

Many of the beliefs and rules in a given family can be traced (using the genogram, for example) to explicit or implicit beliefs and rules learned in the families of origin of the parent(s). Beliefs and rules may have been brought, unexamined, into the new family. Alternatively, partners may have consciously rejected aspects of working models from one or both families of origin and worked to create a new and different set of beliefs and rules for their family life.

It has become clear that there is no one right working model of family beliefs and rules. Different organizational patterns and roles, communication styles, and relationships to the extended family and larger social systems are possible and functional, often based on and embedded in differing ethnic, cultural, or religious practices, beliefs, and worldviews. Particularly where practitioners or researchers are working with families from an ethnic, cultural, or religious background different from their own, a team approach—including a team member who has a background similar to the client family's—is helpful in understanding different but functional beliefs, rules, and practices.

Satir's (1988) work on family rules demonstrates the importance of understanding a family's working model in both assessment and change efforts. This area of family life is also illuminated in recent discussions of individual and family stories and narratives (Holland & Kilpatrick, 1993) and associated family rituals and patterns of extended family gatherings and celebration (Laird, 1984).

The tool of family sculpting, which involves family members dramatically portraying family emotional patterns (as demonstrated and discussed by Peggy Papp, 1974), can be powerfully effective in revealing painful but implicit and unrecognized relationships and rules in the family system. Making visible these emotional relationship patterns and beliefs in a behavioral way can result in family members deciding to let go of outdated working models and create new, more functional, patterns and rules.

Family members can role-play or dramatize new patterns and scenarios, trying them on for size. Some practitioners or families may not feel comfortable with such playacting, and not all methods and tools fit every family. For some families, however, moving beyond intellectual discussion or "just talk" to a more kinesthetic approach—in which they experience behaviorally the rules and patterns governing their family interactions and are helped to practice new roles and communication patterns—can be very effective.

An important premise in the examination of family beliefs and rules is that these are indeed working models. Shared or partially shared internal image systems have developed (consciously or unconsciously) over time in response to external and internal conditions as the family's best solution at the time. The corollary of this view is that current beliefs and rules that guide not only behaviors but also cognitive attitudes and emotional interrelationships are subject to change as new challenges emerge and new information is gained.

An open-ended developmental view is particularly important in the area of family beliefs, rules, rituals, and narratives (Walsh, 1993; White & Epston, 1990). Patterns learned previously—whether in the family of origin or in earlier stages of the current decisionally created family—can be examined and evaluated. New narratives, patterns, and rituals can be created and tried out to replace outdated models. Subsequently, these new working models can be reexamined and reevaluated to meet fresh challenges and cope with changed internal or external circumstances.

Family Communication

Family communication patterns can begin to be seen before the first session begins, in that who calls the agency—and even where family members sit in physical relation to one another at the first meeting—can provide clues to relationships. Does the woman/mother make the first contact? Is it difficult to involve other family members, especially the partner/husband/father in "the problem"? If there are two parents or partners, do they sit together or separately during the first session?

In some families, all or almost all communications about family matters flow through the mother. In other families, the father is the authoritative source of information. In still other couple relationships, authority and information are shared fairly equally. In addition, in some families, children are actively encouraged to speak for themselves and to share their thoughts and feelings, whereas in other families one or both parents consistently speak for other family members, including children and spouse. In some families, a child or children are the spokesperson(s), indicating a reversal of "normal" family roles.

Mattaini (1993) discusses the use of "family diagrams" (p. 45) and "family exchanges" (p. 46) to elucidate strong, tenuous, and stressful relationships between individual members of the family as well as positive and negative communication exchanges. Because of the importance of communication in facilitating all other aspects of family life, assessment of and work on a family's communication skills may be a key initial point of intervention. Assessment should focus on the degree of active listening, abilities in sending clear and congruent messages as well as clarifying incoming messages that are not understood, skills in problem solving through generation of alternatives, and discussion and deliberation aimed toward consensus on choices. Interventions addressing communication skills building in the family may also facilitate family members' ability to negotiate with staff of agencies and other organizational actors in the neighborhood and local social systems.

Family Life Chronology

Based on the developmental view of family life, a family life chronology (Satir, 1983) or family time line can reveal key events in the family's life over time. Figure 3.6 depicts some key events in the life of

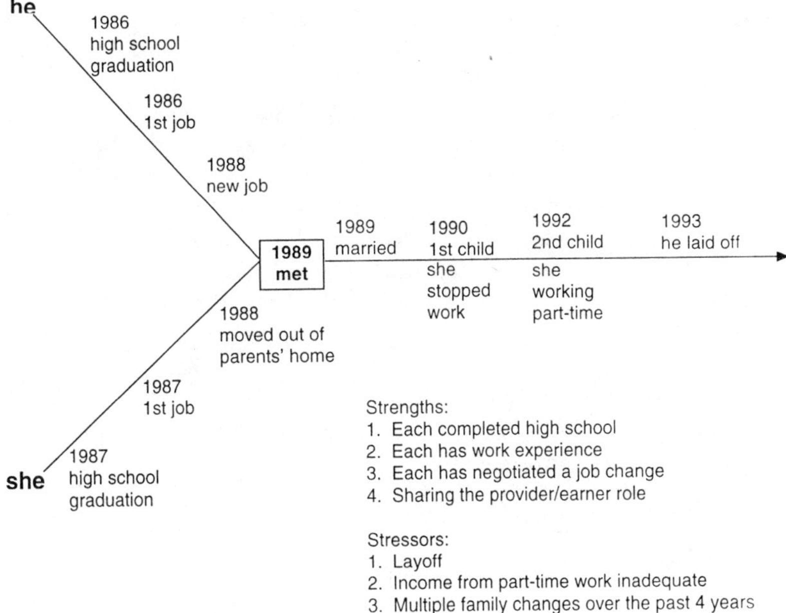

Figure 3.6. Smith Family Time Line

a working-class couple with two preschool children (the time line was created in 1993). Work on the family time line can reveal for the practitioner as well as for family members, combinations of strengths and stressors.

Some strengths for the family depicted in Figure 3.6 include (a) completion of high school by both parents, (b) ability of each parent to function independently as worker and earner, (c) ability of each to negotiate a job change in the past, and (d) the couple's willingness to share the provider role after the birth of children. Stressors include current unemployment of the primary wage earner, inadequate income from one part-time job, and multiple transitions (from single adults, to married couple, to birth of first child, to birth of a second child, and mother's return to work) within a short period of time (4 years).

Along with other tools such as the genogram and ecomap, the family time line can place a "family problem" such as marital conflict in its larger context so that stresses, resources, and meanings can be understood and strategies for intervention and change can be devised. The family time line can be particularly useful in identifying and understanding family system stress and coping around family life cycle transitions. For example, in a family that has experienced stable functioning for a fairly long period of time (e.g., children were launched some years ago, and retirement income has been stable and adequate), a sudden change (heart attack, surgery, or diagnosis of cancer and large medical expenses not covered by Medicare) may be experienced as overwhelming, compared to the background equilibrium. Talking with family members about previous coping successes (e.g., how they coped with their own parents' illnesses and impending deaths; how extended-family members did or did not assist with financial and emotional resources in previous illnesses) may help to reduce initial anxiety, releasing energy for problem solving and mobilizing resources within and outside the family system.

Home Visits

A traditional social work assessment tool in the past has been the home visit. Although its use may not be appropriate in all situations, depending on the agency setting, policy, and the presenting problem, a home visit can yield a rich array of valuable information and can, in some circumstances, enable family members to feel more comfortable in discussing many individual and family problems and issues.

A home visit can prompt a discussion of whether the family's housing is rented or owned, and with or without specific discussion with family members, the worker can observe whether the family lives in a single-family dwelling, trailer, duplex, or multifamily housing unit. External space, including whether there is a yard, and location in the neighborhood can also be observed and commented on if appropriate.

Inside the home, a number of aspects of housing space can be observed and discussed where needed. For example, does the space seem crowded or spacious for the number of people living here? Are rooms and doors open or closed? Are people able to move around easily? An exploration of how long the family has lived in this house or apartment; previous housing arrangements, if any; family members' satisfaction with current housing and internal living arrangements; and their hopes, if any, for different housing in the future may provide clues for understanding aspects of current family stress and strengths.

Discussion of family organizational roles may include such aspects of household maintenance as (a) Who does house cleaning, when, and to whose standard of cleanliness? (b) Is yard work done and, if so, who does it? (c) Who takes care of pets? (d) Who is responsible for repairs and how often are they necessary (depending, e.g., on whether there is a responsible landlord, and on the age of the dwelling and its previous upkeep)? (e) Are there in-home laundry facilities, or must someone go elsewhere to wash clothes? As a part of this discussion, some understanding of daily, weekly, and monthly routines and time and task management demands may emerge as part of current family difficulties.

Observation of spaciousness versus space limitations may assist the social worker *and* family members in understanding aspects of family communication as well as connections with support networks. For example, is there space (and time) for couple discussion and decision making apart from the constant demands of household and children? Is there space (and time) for whole-family discussions that include older children and adolescents (e.g., around a kitchen table or family dinner table)? Does the family eat together and, if so, how often? Are these happy or tense occasions? Is there conversation or does television dominate?

Furthermore, is there enough space to invite other persons into the home—for example, members of the extended-family network, friends (including children's and adolescents' friends), and other members of the family support network (e.g., from a church, religious group, or neighborhood association)? Discussion of family gatherings, ceremonies, and celebrations in the family space can lead to better understandings of both nuclear and extended-family beliefs, rituals, stories, and positive (or negative) connections. Examination of whether outsiders are or can be welcomed may provide important clues to the family system's openness or closedness as well as relationships with neighbors and resource personnel—for example, school teachers, health workers, staff of youth recreation programs, staff of social service agencies—in the neighborhood or local community.

In the midst of these discussions, a social worker or other human service professional—particularly if he or she is from a similar ethnic, religious, cultural, and socioeconomic background to family members —can sense whether the overall atmosphere in this house and home is nurturing or somewhat (or even very) threatening. Such observations and impressions may provide key understandings for assessment and for possible future interventions and change.

Larger Social Systems

For many families and family practitioners today, an understanding of family system functioning must include an ability to discern and assess the impact of and interactions with the policies and organizational structures embedded in multiple levels of larger social systems, including the neighborhood, local community, state, nation, and the socioeconomic system of the globe. Practice tools to assist practitioners and researchers in their assessment of larger systems include (a) the neighborhood walk, (b) data mapping, (c) the context diagram, (d) program evaluations, and (e) policy analysis.

As part of a home visit, the practitioner or researcher has the opportunity to at least drive through the neighborhood in which the family lives. An even better understanding of the family's residential context can be obtained from a *neighborhood walk,* perhaps with at least one family member. During a walking tour of the immediate neighborhood, the social worker can observe such aspects of everyday life as housing stock, distance to schools, retail shopping, laundromats, day care, frail elder care, medical care facilities, recreation facilities for children and youth, social service agencies, and bus or mass transit stops. If the family does not own a reliable automobile, it may be important to explore how the bus and mass transit system are (or are not) tied together and whether riders can easily get around the community for employment; retail shopping; and educational, medical, and social services. Presence or absence of nearby police and fire protection can be observed, and where appropriate, discussion of crime in the area and how safe family members feel walking or driving in their neighborhood can be an important area for understanding. Knowledge of ethnic patterns in the neighborhood as well as the presence and power of neighborhood organizations—from parent-teacher organizations to community action groups to gangs—may be helpful. The neighborhood walk can reveal a more nuanced picture of the family in context in everyday life as stresses and supports for the family as a whole and for particular family members become evident.

As discussed by Mattaini (1993), *data mapping* is a tool for graphically displaying social indicators related to current patterns and changes at the local community level. This involves "mapping community data geographically" (p. 125), and can include pinpointing employment, food and other retail shops, banks, schools, day care and recreation facilities, medical and social service agencies, and public transportation routes and stops. Rates of problems can also be mapped by neighborhood, including poverty, unemployment, unsafe or abandoned housing, school dropout, crime, referrals for child abuse, and infant mortality. In addition, voting patterns and political participation can be delineated. Mapping over time may assist researchers in identifying key factors contributing to community and neighborhood deterioration or revitalization and can help practitioners and agencies in targeting and evaluating services.

At the agency level, practitioners and researchers can engage collaboratively in assessments that include *context diagramming* (see Mattaini, 1993, p. 143) of connections between local agencies and delivery systems. An agency context diagram delineates relationships between the agency and other organizations and actors in the local social system—such as clients; community agencies; community action groups; businesses; education, health, and other service systems; and state and local officials.

Additional tools are needed to enhance workers' ability to perceive and understand program and funding relationships between local and state, local and national, state and national, and public and private organizations and services. Tools are needed for uncovering the impacts of global economic changes on national, state, and local employment and service systems.

Program evaluations and *policy analysis* are steps in these directions, but there is a critical need for tools to put all—or at least many—of these pieces together into more comprehensive and understandable whole pictures. Currently, program evaluations and policy analyses tend to be focused primarily on only one aspect of social services or social problems, such as housing, education, medical care, mental illness, crime, income maintenance, children's services, services for youth, or the elderly. Alternatively, policy analysis and proposed interventions may address service connections at the national, state, or local level, with inadequate thought given to planning for an effective fit with already-existing financing and regulatory interconnections between systems (global, national, state, local, and neighborhood levels).

Social work practitioners, individually and collectively, must become involved in policy practice at multiple social systems levels—through advocacy, lobbying, coalition building, research, and administration of effective programs and services. Social workers and other human service professionals have critical roles to play in developing knowledge that enables all citizens to understand how multilevel social systems work so that voters can make informed decisions regarding new policies and needed changes.

Measurement Tools

Over the past decade, a number of measurement tools have been developed for use by practitioners and researchers in understanding overall family system functioning as well as various aspects of individual family member functioning. These measures can be used to assess family difficulties and to evaluate interventions and change. The development of valid and reliable measures for multiple aspects of family life contributes to ongoing knowledge building for effective social work practice. In this section, I present several family system measures. Then, I identify resources for locating instruments that can be used to assess various individual and family arenas and problems. Last, I discuss a comprehensive measurement package that is currently being used in work with low-income families in a neighborhood-based family service agency.

A number of models with associated measurement instruments have been developed for evaluating family system functioning. Some of these are discussed briefly by Mattaini (1993, pp. 18ff). These include the Olson Circumplex Model and FACES III (Olson, 1986; see also discussion of the Clinical Rating Scale, Thomas & Olson, 1993), the Beavers Model and associated instruments (Beavers & Hampson, 1990), the McMaster Model of Family Functioning (MMFF) and Family Assessment Device (FAD) (Epstein, Baldwin, & Bishop, 1983; Epstein et al., 1982), and the Moos Family Environment Scale (FES) (Moos & Moos, 1986).

A number of rapid assessment instruments (RAIs) have been developed and tested in recent years for use by practitioners in assessing individuals and families and evaluating practice outcomes. Measures for such concepts and problems as self-esteem, depression, and parent-child relationships have been developed and validated by Hudson (1982; see also Nurius & Hudson, 1993). Fischer and Corcoran's (1994) re- view of RAIs for clinical practice includes measures for assessment and work with children, adults, couples, and families (see also Touliatos, Perlmutter, & Straus, 1990). These resources make it more possible for practitioners and researchers to identify common measures for practice evaluation of interventions and change. Agencies and researchers can begin to combine aggregate data from the work done by many clinicians in studies that identify key factors in effective practice with different client systems.

Many of these instruments, however, assume that interventions and change at the individual or family system level will be sufficient to resolve the identified difficulties and problems. Particularly in work with families impacted by stress from larger social systems—such as unemployment, poverty, and lack of access to needed services—a more comprehensive package of assessment measures is needed.

The Appendix presents a set of assessment and follow-up tools and forms currently in use by social workers in a clinical research project with low-income families being served by a neighborhood-based family service center (see also Nair, Blake, & Vosler, in press). Specific types of data are being tracked with families at specified time intervals (intake, 6 months, 1 year, 2 years, and case closing). Data include detailed demographics, a profile of household income and expenses, a general problems checklist, and a systemic (family) patterns checklist. Also being used by staff (with permission) is Taynor, Nelson, and Daugherty's (1990) Family Intervention Scale. Beginning at 6 months, measures have been developed to indicate (a) social work methods used, (b) systemic interventions used, and (c) client satisfaction.

Agency staff in this project are involved in community development and programming activities including neighborhood needs assessments, program planning and implementation—such as family life education, child care, and before- and after-school individualized care (BASIC). As staff work with family members having difficulties in larger social systems (such as relationships with the housing board, town council, school, police, etc.), staff members are able to identify problems and issues that emerge across groupings of families. The agency then engages in research and advocacy around problems that affect these groups of client families. (For a description of a successful collaborative effort to improve housing policy at the national level, see Vosler & Nair, 1993.) This project is an initial effort to identify and measure the many factors that are thought to be relevant for understanding effective work with stressed low-income families. One of the project's unique strengths is that it incorporates into knowledge building information regarding the impact on family functioning of stress from larger social systems.

ENGAGING MULTIPLE FAMILY MEMBERS

Systemic practice focuses not only on individual family members but more specifically on relationships between two or more family members as well as on relationships between the family and larger social systems and structures. To understand current family patterns and relationships, social workers and other human service practitioners need skills in engaging multiple family members in both assessment and intervention. Family engagement skills are used to involve family members who may be reluctant participants, such as partners, husbands, fathers, adolescent children, and extended-family members.

In the United States today, the woman/mother continues to be seen as the family member primarily responsible for child care and child rearing. (In Chapter 4, I summarize empirical findings in this regard.) An individualistic cultural worldview, or working model of beliefs and rules (Bellah et al., 1985) sends messages to the woman/mother that if there are problems in the family it is her responsibility to get individual help in getting things "fixed." As a result, practitioners may need to expend considerable time and energy in convincing the person who first approaches the agency for help that involvement by all family members in interviews and interventions may be a key to problem resolution and change.

Once the practitioner has been successful in bringing together multiple family members, skills in conducting and managing the family interview will be key. An interview with multiple participants is different from one-on-one interviews in important ways, including content and often intensity. Family practitioners have found that effective use of family interview time often involves a team approach, as well as videotaping of interviews. One or more practitioners behind a one-way mirror observe the family being interviewed and may make recommendations to the in-session worker. Alternatively, team members may later view a videotape and discuss observations with the primary worker. The team member's specific role is to track communication and other interaction patterns between family members, between the worker and individuals, and between the worker and the family group as a whole.

Such an approach requires an agency setting in which there is space for a family interview with multiple members (and quiet toys or books for younger children when they tire of listening to adults and older children talking). It also requires commitment by the agency to specialized equipment such as a one-way mirror and videotaping and viewing facilities. Time is also required for staff to participate in the team; to view and analyze videotapes; and to participate in case discussions, feedback, consultation, and continuing staff development.

The advantage of engaging multiple family members includes seeing the problem from various viewpoints for a more comprehensive picture.

Studies have shown that family members often differ in their perceptions of family life and functioning (Green & Vosler, 1992; Kolevzon, Green, Fortune, & Vosler, 1988). In addition, family members who have been involved from the outset are more likely to participate in change efforts.

In an interview with multiple family members, an advantage of the team approach is the ability to observe actual family interaction patterns. The in-session practitioner manages the interview process while a behind-the-mirror team member focuses on observation of family interaction and content.

UNDERSTANDING DIVERSITY THROUGH TEAM CONSULTATION

Related to the team concept is the practice strategy of team consultation. As demonstrated by the previous discussion of assessment tools, in work with families an almost overwhelming amount of data can be generated. Such data are needed to understand comprehensively and work effectively with the family in context. No individual practitioner can be expected—or can expect of herself or himself—to have practice expertise in all areas of family life and problems. For example, the team that developed the General Problems Checklist shown in the Appendix identified over 50 potential problem areas. They include such diverse problems as marital conflict, extramarital relationships, spousal abuse, physical and sexual abuse of children, unstable housing, deficient nutrition, conflict with an employer, low skills for employment, acute or chronic medical problems, mental illness, learning disabilities, suicide, substance and alcohol abuse, and gambling. If the practitioner team and family agree that the difficulties include problems in a specialized area and team members are not trained in that particular area, both the team and the family can benefit from consultations with a practitioner skilled in the problem area.

With increased professional awareness of the importance of understanding family diversity, agencies that build staff teams that include both women and men and persons from different ethnic backgrounds can enrich staff understandings of family meanings and beliefs and enhance teams' ability to assess and intervene effectively. Literature on work with families from diverse backgrounds is available (see Boyd-Franklin, 1989, 1993; Ellman & Taggart, 1993; McGoldrick, 1993;

McGoldrick, Pearce, & Giordano, 1982). Beyond familiarity with the literature, a team that includes a member from an ethnic background similar to the client family can (a) enhance the initial joining process with the family, (b) yield important in-session insights, and (c) expand other team members' awareness and skills. (For further discussion of cultural and gender meanings and associated socioeconomic contexts, see Waldegrave, 1990.)

Either on staff or as part of ongoing consultation, teams in agencies working with families need access to expertise on diverse family issues. Consultation ongoing or as needed might include assistance in work with various income and SES groups (e.g., families facing role overload from employed work and family work, unemployment, or poverty); unmarried mothers; teenage parents; divorced or divorcing families, including single-parent households and remarriage families; and special issues for gay and lesbian families, families in later life, and families dealing with chronic illness or disability. In each of these areas, consultant expertise, based on knowledge of current theory and research, can be invaluable in providing to the team ways to understand current family functioning as well as access to intervention models that have been demonstrated as effective.

INTERVENING AND EVALUATING

Because of the complexity and diversity of family social systems, it is obvious that no single intervention model or set of practice principles is sufficient to guide practice with every client family. Several empirically oriented intervention models have been developed and have been shown to be effective with some families. These include the Olson Circumplex Model (Olson, 1986), the Beavers Model (Beavers & Hampson, 1990), and the McMaster Model of Family Functioning (MMFF; Epstein et al., 1982). These models, along with various family therapy approaches (such as those developed by Bowen, Satir, Minuchin, Haley, Whitaker, and a host of other seminal practitioners), focus change efforts on the family system and on family members and dyads or triads in the family. (See Walsh, 1993, for a comparison of a number of these models.)

Little attention has been directed to interventions and evaluation of change in larger systems that support—or fail to support—family functioning and efforts for change. The staff of the agency research project using the evaluation instruments delineated in the Appendix incorporate in their assessment and intervention planning a *dual* focus. This includes intrafamily systemic interventions (see Systemic Interventions Checklist) and more traditional social casework methods (see Social Work Methods Used checklist) that link family members with services in the neighborhood or local community systems. It must be emphasized, however, that this agency is in a national social system that has very low unemployment, excellent transportation systems, effective housing policies, and neighborhood-based affordable health care and other social services. In addition, where problems are identified, agency staff see it as their professional responsibility to identify links between family-level difficulties and larger-system functioning, and subsequently to devise, recommend, and plan for needed policy changes at local or national levels (see Vosler & Nair, 1993).

In many parts of the United States, where policies are not as supportive of families and programs may not be in place to help family members cope with stress from external systems, there is a need for collaborative practice research to identify and track changes in (a) family demographics and problems, (b) resources that are realistically available, accessible, and affordable to the family—and therefore also gaps in the delivery system—and (c) structures and processes in larger systems that negatively impact on family functioning. Such larger system structures and processes include plant closings; high unemployment rates; high neighborhood crime rates; high absentee landlord and housing deterioration rates; inaccessible transportation systems; and the movement of retail shops, education, and other services out of the neighborhood or local area. Over time, such data can provide to staff, especially in neighborhood-based agencies, (a) an understanding of interactions among families, services, and larger-system structures; (b) a means of evaluating outcomes of programs and services at multiple levels, including individual family members, family system functioning, and neighborhood and community functioning; and (c) empirically based theory both for shifting consensus within larger systems and for advocating new and potentially effective approaches, policies, and programs.

In this model, professional practice becomes focused not only on work with individuals and families but on understanding that microsystem work can be effective only when neighborhood and wider systems support and enhance family functioning. Macro work must include analysis of policies and programs at local, state, and national levels and must provide ways to modify and develop new policies and programs. Areas for modification include funding streams, the functioning of economic systems, and regulations and incentives. The encouragement and development of leadership, political participation, and activism become critical components of practice. Equally important, educational work in the community with individuals and groups representing the diversity of the local community becomes important in identifying common beliefs and building consensus on needed economic and social programs and services. (See Jansson, 1994, for further discussion of policy practice strategies and skills.)

MULTILEVEL SOCIAL SYSTEMS KNOWLEDGE BUILDING AND CHANGE

It is clear that social workers have access to large amounts of data regarding individuals, families, and the functioning of larger social systems, both from their individual practice experiences and from information systems at agency and larger-system levels. The work of comprehensive knowledge building regarding the interactions and interconnections between multiple levels of social systems as well as the work of testing the effectiveness of varying practice models for different populations and problems has only recently begun on a fairly wide scale.

For knowledge to be developed, valid and reliable measures for a variety of indicators at multiple systems levels are needed. At least some commonalties are needed in key concepts and their operationalization, so that findings can be compared and contrasted across programs, problems, and populations.

Until recently, knowledge building has too often been confined to a few highly specialized professional researchers or to academicians in psychology, anthropology, sociology, economics, and political science. Increasingly, social workers—including direct service and policy practitioners along with agency administrators and researchers—must face the challenge of developing new ways of engaging in professional practice. This must include (a) use of currently available theories and practice models for identifying key factors in systems functioning at multiple levels (including the individual, the family, and larger systems), (b) assessing and specifying components for intervention and change at each appropriate system level, and (c) evaluating both process and outcomes at multiple levels.

This knowledge building necessarily involves a variety of participants as actors, as changes in social systems entail shifts in rules and roles and at times require transformations in common beliefs and working models as well. Communication and consensus-building skills are needed because (a) understanding and describing current functioning, (b) devising plans for interventions and change, and (c) evaluating both process and outcomes involves not only social workers at a variety of levels but also client families, colleagues from a variety of research disciplines, staff personnel associated with a range of relevant social agencies and organizations, business persons, politicians, advocacy groups, and a variety of fellow citizens.

SUMMARY

Multilevel systemic family practice requires tools and methods for assessing and working with families in the context of larger social systems. Assessment tools include the multigenerational genogram, the household ecomap, intrafamily mapping, household income-expenses assessment, discussion of family beliefs and rules, observation of family communication patterns, a family life chronology or time line, home visits, a neighborhood walk, local community data mapping, agency context diagramming, program evaluations, and policy analysis. Methods include skills in engaging and working with families in interviews with multiple family members—often using a team approach, use of team consultation, development and use of valid and reliable family and larger-systems measures, and evaluation of practice for ongoing multilevel social systems knowledge building and change.

In the remainder of this book, I address theory and current research findings as well as tools and models for practice and knowledge building in several key areas in which changes or structural gaps in larger social systems have been shown to impact family life negatively. These are (a) current normative stress from work-family role overload (Chapters 4 and 5), (b) potentially catastrophic stress from unemployment (Chapters 6 and 7), and (c) stress pileup from chronic poverty (Chapters 8 and 9). Case examples are provided at the beginning of Chapters 5, 7, and 9.

Chapter 4

FAMILIES AND WORK
Theory and Research

In this chapter, I review current social science knowledge regarding family coping with changes in "employed work" and "family work." Stress from multiple roles and potential role overload has recently become "normative" in the United States, particularly among families with children and other dependents. First, a brief overview sets theory and research in this area in historical perspective. Next, I delineate theoretical models, concepts, and definitions. A review of current research findings follows, including special attention to diversity in family structural forms and unique stressors. Finally, I offer a critique of current research, pointing out limitations and knowledge gaps, and briefly discuss implications for social work practice, indicating directions for professional involvement in knowledge building and work at multiple systems levels.

HISTORY OF THEORY AND RESEARCH

A historical review of theory and research in the area of families and work reveals that until recently family and work—that is, participation in the paid labor force—were considered two separate spheres with roles assigned by gender (Gerstel & Gross, 1987; Piotrkowski, Rapoport, & Rapoport, 1987). Beginning in the 1940s, increasing numbers of women entered the paid labor force. Research at that time focused on the assumed deleterious consequences of maternal employment for families, especially children. Over the past two decades, as structural economic changes have resulted in more and more families requiring two paychecks to remain in the middle class—or even to make ends meet—studies have focused on role overload from previously "invisible" family work. Calls for political changes at multiple levels—affordable child care, parental leave, flexible work schedules—have emerged. Connections between various streams of research and common concepts and theoretical frameworks have only recently begun to be developed, however.

Separate Spheres

As Gerstel and Gross (1987, p. 8) point out, with industrial capitalism came "the temporal, normative, and spatial separation of jobs and family," with men expected to participate in the labor force and women assigned to the private—and therefore to social science research relatively invisible—sphere of the family. Women were expected to maintain the household, raise children, and provide support for their husbands' careers. Support included emotional nurturing, relocation of the family if required by the company, and in some cases social entertainment for the husbands' coworkers and their spouses (see Voydanoff, 1988, p. 3).

Thompson and Walker (1991, p. 81) point out that all along an additional invisible reality has been the labor force participation of women with children who had to find employment to provide basic necessities for their families. In particular, because of racial discrimination and economic barriers for African American men, wage work has historically been necessary for large numbers of African American women (Harley, 1990).

Recent research has documented the previously relatively invisible community work and multiple nonfamily roles of women in the 1950s—in households where husbands were professionals as well as in nonprofessional households. The number of these public roles was found to be positively related to mothers' self-esteem and general life satisfaction (Miller, Moen, & Dempster-McClain, 1991). An additional reality that has been largely invisible in the separate spheres framework is fathers' participation in the unpaid sphere of family work (Barnett & Baruch, 1988).

Thus, although a prevailing and traditional social science working model of assumptions and beliefs has viewed work as the man's domain and family as the woman's (his wife's) responsibility (see, e.g., Parsons

& Bales, 1955), all along there have been invisible exceptions to this supposed reality of gendered separate spheres.

Maternal Employment

In the 1960s and 1970s, increasing numbers of social science researchers began to focus on the large numbers of employed mothers in U.S. society and on possible deleterious consequences of this trend for families (Voydanoff, 1988). In particular, the impact of maternal employment on children was of concern. It is interesting to note that paternal employment has seldom if ever been seen as a potential social problem, although paternal *un*employment has been and continues to be viewed as problematic.

Early studies showed that in comparison with women who were exclusively housewives, employed women were *less* psychologically distressed (for a review, see Mirowsky & Ross, 1989, p. 86). At about the same time, other researchers were finding that day care in high-quality centers for preschool children did *not* result in harm for children's physical, mental, and psychological development (see Belsky, 1990). An interesting question for empirical exploration is whether these findings helped to shift the beliefs of individuals and families—as well as social consensus in larger systems—toward increasing acceptance of mothers' participation in the paid labor force. Often lost to view, as Belsky points out, has been the fact that the purchase of high-quality preschool child care was affordable primarily for professional middle-class or higher-wage dual-career families; the findings are not generalizable to all children of employed mothers.

Role Stress

Structural changes in the economy over the past two decades have decreased many men's earning power and resulted in increasing numbers of families with young children having to rely on two rather than only one worker-earner (Voydanoff, 1988; Wilkie, 1991). In the 1980s, numbers of studies have focused on role overload in dual-earner families (Aldous, 1982; Eckenrode & Gore, 1990; Pleck, 1985; Pleck & Staines, 1985; Voydanoff, 1987). These studies have begun to make visible previously invisible unpaid family work. This research has established that the majority of "second-shift" family work is performed by women (Hochschild, 1989; Menaghan & Parcel, 1991). Findings from these studies are reviewed in detail later in this chapter.

Concomitant with these changes in sociocultural beliefs and socioeconomic structures have been increasing calls for political changes. Such changes need to address the realities of maternal employment and role overload to enable parents to cope with balancing family and job responsibilities. Some policies regarding child care and maternity leave have been enacted by Congress at the national level, affecting states, local communities, and employers. At the same time, the controversy over whether every AFDC mother should be required to become a full-time earner reflects a continuing ambivalence among citizens and policymakers over the role paid employment should play in the lives of parents, particularly mothers (see, e.g., Chilman, 1993; Ellwood, 1988; Moen, 1992).

In summary, social science research to date has documented that increasing numbers of women with young children are in the labor force. Some of these families are coping well and their members—adults and children—are physically and psychologically healthy and satisfied with their lives. On the other hand, many women—particularly those who are mothers of young children—struggle to balance employed work and family work. Often, these mothers have little or no assistance from their spouses or the fathers of their children. To understand how best to work with families struggling with these issues, social work practitioners and other human service professionals need concepts and theories that make visible both stressors and potential solutions within multiple social systems.

CONCEPTS, DEFINITIONS, AND THEORETICAL FRAMEWORKS

In recent reviews, Piotrkowski et al. (1987) and Voydanoff (1988) have utilized social systems and stress and coping theoretical frameworks in understanding research findings regarding families and work. Piotrkowski et al. (1987) conclude their literature review by discussing three frameworks that have emerged as salient in the arena of families and work: (a) families as "complex social systems" (p. 272); (b) a family "developmental framework" (p. 273)—that is, the family life cycle (or "career") view—emphasizing normative transitions and tasks in the work-family relationship; and (c) "family stress theory" (p. 274), including catastrophic and chronic stressors. Voydanoff (1988) incorporates these theoretical frameworks and calls for an "expanded conceptualization of work and family" (p. 10) that focuses on (a) multiple social systems levels—including understandings of organizations at the local community level and the structure of the economy at the national level—and (b) the continuing importance of gender and gendered roles in U.S. society.

To explicate the complex relationships between families and work implied by these theoretical frameworks, the following concepts are discussed in some detail: (a) dual-earner and dual-career families, (b) employed work and family work in the family social system, (c) task accomplishment versus a manager subrole within the task performance of particular family organizational roles, and (d) role overload.

Dual-Earner and Dual-Career Families

Early studies tended to focus on *dual-career* families, or "two-career couples in which both husbands and wives are employed in professional or managerial occupations" (Voydanoff, 1988, pp. 2-3; see, e.g., Kanter, 1977). Recent research has established, however, that "over half of two-parent families with dependent children are now '*dual-earner*' families . . . in which [both] husbands and wives are gainfully employed [italics added]" (Piotrkowski et al., 1987, p. 254). Piotrkowski et al. also note that dual-career households "may [now] be a 'minor variant' of dual-earner families" (p. 272).

The important distinction that needs to be made between dual-earner and dual-career families is that for many U.S. families in the 1990s—particularly households with children or other dependents—having *both* parents working may well be not a *choice* but a *necessity.* Within the general descriptive category of dual-earner families—that is, families in which both parents are in the labor force—there is a subcategory of dual-career families for whom participation in employed work is seen as a career, with each parent committed to his or her job as an important part of participation in society outside of the family. As Schwartz and Scott (1994, p. 300) point out, a career implies (a) "extensive training, usually a college or professional degree," (b) "specific paths of upward mobility," and (c) "commitment beyond a 9-5 workday."

These distinctions alert practitioners and researchers to the importance of understanding differing kinds of families. For example, how much choice do family members actually have in their employed-work role(s)—that is, is the family a dual-earner family by necessity or by choice? Furthermore, to what extent do individual career goals complement or conflict with family life—that is, to what extent is this a dual-career couple and how do the two careers fit with family roles and tasks? Finally, based on larger-system constraints as well as family beliefs and understandings, what kinds of changes in the work-family balance are possible for the family as a whole and for individual family members?

Employed Work and Family Work

Early research focusing on separate spheres differentiated families from work, implying that unpaid household and child-rearing activities were not work (Piotrkowski et al., 1987, p. 254; Piotrkowski & Hughes, 1993, p. 191). Much of the economics literature has exacerbated this tendency to render family work invisible by designating all activities outside of the wage labor market—except necessary time for eating and sleeping—as leisure. This view implies that the only two important choices individuals have are (a) work in the labor force or (b) leisure time (Baumol & Blinder, 1991, p. 428).

As Voydanoff (1988, p. 12) points out, consideration of *both* paid work—or employed work—*and* unpaid work in the household—or family work—is vital to researchers' and practitioners' understanding of families in their efforts to cope with the complex stresses of multiple activities and tasks. Family work includes a variety of roles. One of these intrafamily roles is the provider role, also termed the breadwinner, wage earner, or worker-earner role. A number of additional family roles must be performed for family members to become and remain organized as a social system that functions in healthy ways. These include roles of family leadership and decision making, household maintenance, dependents' care, and supervision and socialization of children and youth.

The role of family leadership and decision making involves time and energy committed to communication. Through ongoing interaction, family members develop a sense of cohesion as well as creating working models of the family's beliefs and rules for living. This role also involves developing patterns of communication with extended family members, with friends and coworkers on the job(s), and in religious and other community groups.

The role of household maintenance includes a variety of specific tasks, such as food shopping, meal preparation and cleanup, household cleaning and sanitation, shopping for clothing, laundry, mending, automobile and home repairs, and yard work. Each additional dependent family member is likely to add to the amount of time and energy required to accomplish many of the household maintenance tasks.

Dependents' care can involve time and energy expended in family work with very young, frail elderly, and sick or disabled family members. One or more family members may need to be involved in arranging medical appointments and transportation, preparing specific types of meals, purchasing and maintaining special equipment, carrying out extra sanitation or other procedures, and development of new patterns of communication and interaction among all family members.

Child-rearing and youth supervision and socialization roles incorporate a variety of tasks that emerge and change over the life cycle of the family. Based on the family's working model(s) for family life, decisions must be made regarding infant care; parent-child interactions; family lifestyles; nonparental child care; schooling; before- and after-school and extracurricular activities; sick care; summer activities and supervision; and children's and youths' participation in shaping and reshaping family cohesion and boundaries, roles and organizational structures, rules and beliefs, and communication patterns.

As depicted in Figure 4.1, where both parents participate in employed work—whether by choice or necessity—the family as a social system must develop patterns within a family working model for allocating time and energy to activities involved *both* in the employed work of each *and* in the family work of maintaining the household, developing family leadership, caring for dependents, and rearing children to adulthood. Family working models can incorporate a variety of beliefs, preferences, expectations, and rules for living, but the working model and implied role enactments need to be stable enough for family members to fulfill all of their necessary tasks and experience some sense of well-being and accomplishment.

Task Accomplishment Versus Manager

An additional set of concepts that has emerged from recent research regarding family work are *task accomplishment* versus a *manager* subrole in a variety of family roles. Task accomplishment involves the completion of certain activities, such as cooking dinner, putting a child to bed, or bathing a frail elderly parent. In addition, however, researchers have identified previously invisible manager subroles that involve not only doing—or "helping" with—tasks but also taking responsibility for the ongoing enactment of all of the activities required for successful role performance.

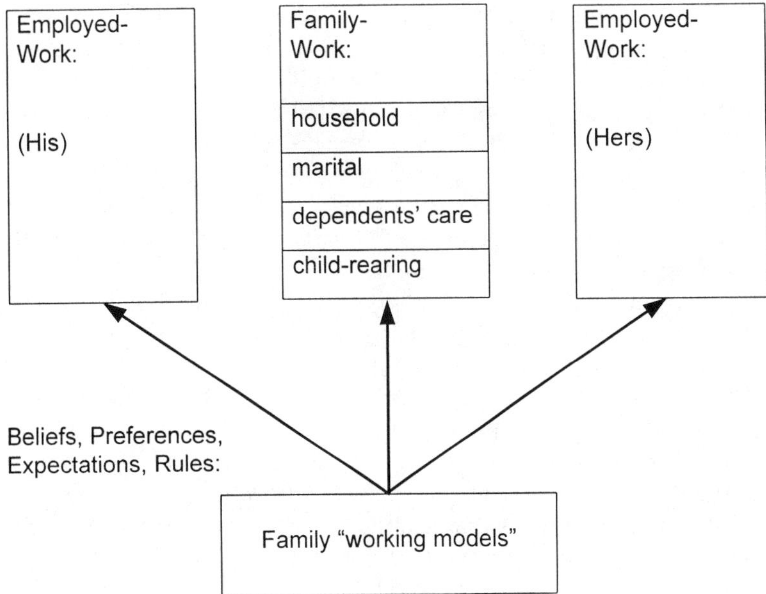

Figure 4.1. Family System Equilibrium

Barnett and Baruch (1988, p. 72), in a study of family work, discuss "responsibility" as "remembering, planning, and scheduling" the multitude of specific tasks necessary for maintaining a household and parenting children. Mederer (1993), in a study of the household maintenance role, found empirical support for differentiating between task accomplishment—such as going grocery shopping or doing laundry—versus the household management role—to "make sure things are ready for the next day," "decide on standards of cleanliness," and "assign chores" (p. 139).

As both specific tasks and the managerial subroles in various family work roles have become more visible, it is clear that organizing and managing even a relatively small family social system can be a time- and energy-consuming enterprise. Even for families who can afford to purchase services that accomplish such tasks as house cleaning or child care, the management of these services is still necessary.

Role Overload

One of the most salient concepts in the literature on the relationship between employed work and family work is that of *role overload.* Schwartz and Scott (1994) define role overload as "a situation in which a person's various roles carry more responsibilities than that person can reasonably manage" (p. 303). As Kelly and Voydanoff (1985) point out, parents' multiple roles in employed work and family work imply demands of time, energy, and commitment; overload occurs when "there is a greater number of prescribed activities than an individual can handle adequately or comfortably" (p. 368).

Employed mothers are particularly vulnerable to role overload. With reference to Figure 4.1, in the family work roles women tend to carry more of the managerial responsibilities as well as spend more time in task accomplishment than other family members. Thus, mothers with small children who are employed full-time are often subject to role overload from trying to fulfill the requirements of two full-time jobs: full-time employed work and full-time family work.

Even when family income permits the purchase of services to supplement task accomplishment in particular areas of family work—such as house cleaning, yard work, or child care—a manager is needed to coordinate and take responsibility for the ongoing operation of all aspects of the extensions of the family work system. Figure 4.2 represents an ecomap of various family and community components that often must fit together in a coordinated family-work system. Only when all of the pieces fit can both parents remain employed. As this ecomap reveals and Voydanoff (1988) discusses in her literature review, the stable availability of accessible and affordable nonparental child care—or frail elder care—in the community social system is essential.

The quality, accessibility, and affordability of nonparental care often depends on the operation of regulations, incentives, or subsidies provided by larger systems, including state and national policies and programs. In some families, extended-family members may be able to provide stable low-cost child care and sick care. But with families scattered across geographic distances, a number of healthy elders needing to be in the labor force to make ends meet, and illness or disability precluding some grandparents' taking on responsibilities for adult children's household maintenance or child care, the African American proverb, "It takes a whole village to raise a child" (McAdoo, 1993, pp. 14-15) becomes an important guiding image for understanding employed work and family work interfacing.

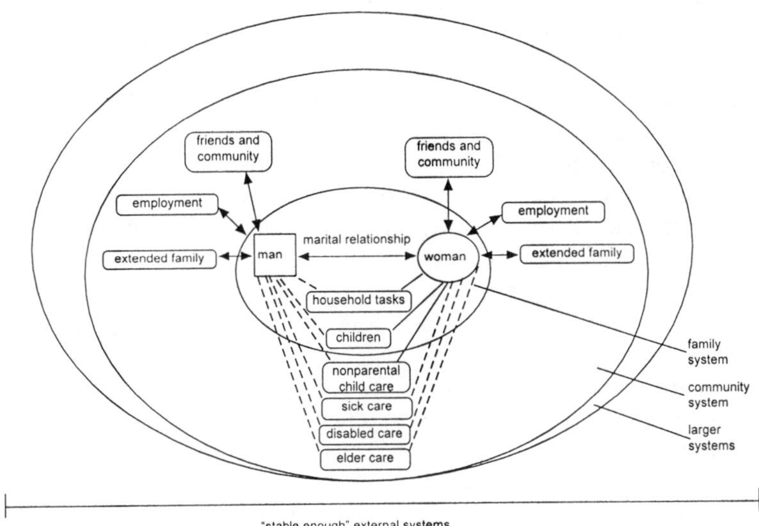

Figure 4.2. Ecomap: Roles and Potential Role Overload

Stress and coping theory highlights the importance of resources, definitions, and beliefs in understanding families' struggles with increased demands and resulting potential for stress pileup and role overload. A first step is making visible the various roles: Who is responsible for which components of those roles—managing versus performing tasks—and the time, energy, and expertise needed to fulfill each of the roles. Help with the identification, marshaling, and organizing of all available supports and resources may in some families be sufficient to relieve role overload. In other cases, the development of stable new resources may be necessary.

Where resources are available but are not being utilized, work with the family regarding beliefs and preferences for work and gendered roles may be needed. Work with the family might also focus on trying out new ways of thinking about lifestyles and activities. The goal with the family might be creative and healthy shifts in the family's working model for balancing the provider role with other family work roles.

The developmental life cycle approach to families as social systems makes clear that adaptation and change are essential in healthy family system functioning. The role enactments that are successful for a newly married couple—for example, that both partners are employed full-time and, based on the beliefs and rules from both families of origin, she does almost all of the housework—may need to be radically rearranged after the birth of their first child. If a child is disabled or chronically ill, different arrangements may need to be negotiated. As children move into school, they may be able to help with some of the housework.

Most youth require at least some peer activities and supervision. In a community where parents and community leaders are linked by common beliefs and cooperative programming, parents may be able to share parenting responsibilities with the wider adult community. Where there are no stable, healthy community structures, however, drugs, guns, violence, and fear can often overwhelm all members of the neighborhood social system.

A family in midlife may have both partners engaged in stable employed work by choice. On the other hand, illness or disability in the parent of a partner may necessitate a sometimes painful rethinking of priorities and role responsibilities.

Voydanoff (1988, p. 7) discusses the "work/family life cycle," pointing to the need for families to construct and reconstruct working models of both role staging and role allocation. For example, will there be a "primary provider" and a "secondary provider," or will this be a "dual-career couple"? If one person is the "secondary provider," what additional role responsibilities will each partner carry?

As Piotrkowski et al. (1987) point out, these patterns are enacted within the constraints and opportunities of larger social systems. For example, young low-income parents may be caught in a "'life-cycle squeeze' in which earnings are not adequate to meet the economic needs created by children" (p. 273). As stress and coping theory indicates, at each transition point there are vulnerabilities and opportunities that must be confronted for the family to function as a healthy but often changing social system.

CURRENT RESEARCH FINDINGS

With these essential concepts—dual earner/dual career, employed work/family work, manager/task accomplishment, and role overload—as a base, I present a summary of findings from the current empirical research literature. This overview is organized under three headings: (a) macrolevel resources and constraints, (b) role allocations and family system outcomes, and (c) family member outcomes—including mothers, fathers, and children.

Macrolevel Resources and Constraints

Specific impacts on a variety of families from structural changes in the U.S. national economy are only beginning to be studied. It is already clear, however, that "a minimum level of economic resources and security is necessary for family formation and stability" (Voydanoff, 1988, p. 4). With rapid declines in the number of high-wage manufacturing jobs in the United States—a trend some have referred to as *deindustrialization* (Wallace & Rothschild, 1988)—and their replacement with lower-wage, often part-time or temporary jobs in the services sector, many families must now have two wage earners to fulfill the requirements of the provider role. Schwartz and Scott (1994) dramatically summarize this trend: "In the 1950s, the goods and services a family needed could be supplied in most cases by the efforts of one wage earner. . . . For a majority of families today, obtaining similar goods and services requires wages from both spouses" (p. 434). It can no longer be assumed that both parents are in the labor force by choice. Increasingly, many households with dependents are dual-earner families by necessity.

Whether by choice or necessity, increasing numbers of mothers of young children are wage earners. Menaghan and Parcel (1991, p. 362) trace a pattern of (a) increasing labor force participation by older married women between 1940 and 1960, (b) increasing participation by mothers of school-aged children in the 1960s and 1970s, and (c) recent increases—to 54% by 1986—in the labor force participation of married women with children under the age of 6. Belsky (1990, p. 895) notes that the labor force participation rate for mothers with an infant under the age of one year is now 51%. Moen (1992) reports that 59% of women with preschool children (p. 14) and 60% of mothers of 2-year-olds (p. 15) are now employed. Balancing employed work and family work has become a normative task for a majority of families with children in the U.S. national social system. Furthermore, wives and mothers are contributing substantially to total family income—providing 31% of family earnings in husband-wife families overall and 39% "when both spouses work full-time year-round" (Spitze, 1991, p. 389).

Although much more research is needed to understand the linkages between macroeconomic shifts and parents' employment patterns, it is clear that at least for the near future, the majority of women—whether they are mothers or not—are now more firmly attached to the labor market (Menaghan & Parcel, 1991). Questions of whether employers as well as structures in larger social systems—including communities, states, and the nation—are or should be supportive of family work realities need to be raised by both professionals and family members as citizens. New social realities of dual-earner families may require changed working models of beliefs and policies at multiple systems levels.

Role Allocations and Family System Outcomes

As women have increasingly moved into employed work, studies have consistently demonstrated that wives continue to do much more family work than husbands. In their literature review, Thompson & Walker (1991) conclude, "Women do three times as many domestic tasks as men" (p. 86) and note that although men engage in family work mostly on weekends, "Women do family work on weekdays *and* weekends" (p. 86). They also note, "Most women and men agree that women should be responsible for family work, and men should 'help out' " (p. 85). In addition, "Mothers, regardless of whether they are employed, carry 90% of the burden of *responsibility* for child care; they plan, organize, delegate, supervise, and schedule" (p. 87). Thus, women—including employed women—carry most of the burden not only for task accomplishment but also for the manager subrole in the performance of a variety of family work roles.

Researchers have examined whether, in recent years, the burden of family work is being shared more equally between men and women. Findings are inconclusive. In one study, researchers found that husbands' share of family work has increased from 20% to 30%; in another study, it appeared that the time husbands' spent in doing household work and child care did not change over a 10-year period (Thompson & Walker, 1991). According to another study, a small number of husbands shared equally with their wives in family work; these families had many—usually young—children and the wives held full-time jobs (Thompson & Walker, 1991).

Thompson and Walker (1991) also note that women tend to do family work that is "unrelenting, repetitive, and routine," whereas men tend to do more infrequent tasks, such as "household repairs, taking out the trash, mowing the lawn, yard work, and gardening" (p. 86). Moreover, "Both women and men experience boredom, fatigue, and tension when they do household work alone" (p. 86).

In a recent study, Blair and Lichter (1991), using a national data set, found that males spent an average of 14 hours per week in "household labor" whereas females spent an average of 33 hours per week. This implies an average family work week of 47 hours. The authors also found that household tasks—such as meal preparation, cleaning house, outdoor tasks, auto maintenance, shopping, and so forth—were highly segregated by gender. There was a tendency for couples in which the female was more highly educated to have somewhat decreased gender segregation of tasks.

In an examination of fathers' involvement in parenting tasks and responsibilities, Lamb (1987) argues that four factors are critical in understanding varying degrees of participation: (a) motivation, (b) skills and self-confidence, (c) support, and (d) institutional practices. He argues that societal attitudes and structures often reflect an underlying social assumption, or working model, of beliefs that "Men are first and foremost workers and breadwinners, whereas women are primarily nurturers" (p. 22). Related to this is the extent to which both partners in a family hold this assumption as a working model for their own family; or, alternatively, whether the shared family belief is that mothers and fathers are equally responsible for child rearing. Lamb (1987) further argues that even when both institutional practices and other family members are supportive of increased involvement of the father in parenting, there must be both individual motivation and the requisite skills and self-confidence for child-rearing tasks to be performed on a consistent basis and for the child care manager role to be equally shared.

Few if any family researchers have focused on the need for a *mother* to experience support from institutional practices and other family members, a sense of motivation, and requisite skills and self-confidence to competently carry out *her* parenting role.

Recent research has identified both husbands' and wives' attitudes or preferences, and the match between preferences and actual life situations, as important factors in understanding role allocation and role overload for individuals and families. If both spouses participate in the provider role through employed work, "whether or not the family makes adjustments to reduce any resulting over-load will depend on how it views her labour" (Spitze, 1991, p. 387)—that is, whether family beliefs and preferences define her employment as "a privilege or a necessity, a contribution to the family or a cost" (p. 387). In addition, among married women, "employment was associated with lower distress when it matched individual preferences. Wives' distress was least when they were employed and preferred to be so; of the two possible mismatches, wives' distress was highest when they were not employed but wished they were" (Menaghan & Parcel, 1991, p. 367).

Thompson and Walker (1991) report, "It is not overwork or exhaustion that is the source of discontent among wives; it is inequity" (p. 89). Thompson (1991) notes, "Although most women do more than two thirds of family work, less than a third of these wives feel that this is unfair and want their husbands to contribute more" (p. 182). On the other hand, Blair and Johnson (1992) found in a recent study, using data from the 1988 National Survey of Families and Households, that predictors of perceptions of fairness differed for employed versus nonemployed wives. These findings lend some support to Thompson and Walker's (1991) suggestion, "We will not understand the distribution of domestic work by gender until we know more about the complex meanings of paid and family work for women and men and how partners change or maintain the gendered distribution of work through their daily interactions" (p. 88). An understanding of distributions of employed work and family work in families may need to include not only who does what but also partners' and overall family internal working models —including beliefs, expectations, preferences, and rules.

Concern has emerged over the impact of role changes and role overloads on marital satisfaction and stability. Bumpass (1990) found negative impacts on marital quality when one or more of the following conditions were present: (a) spousal disagreement over the wife's employment—especially if the husband did not want the wife to work, but she was in fact employed; (b) the wife spent more than 45 hours per week in employed work; and (c) "either spouse works on a job where the shift varies" (p. 491). In addition, "Females who regard the division [of household task allocation] as unfair are much more likely to report trouble in their marriage" (p. 491). On the other hand, Spitze (1991) concludes, "Recent studies based on large national samples have reported no effects of wife's employment, occupational commitment or higher occupational status on the reported marital satisfaction of either husband or wife" (p. 384). In a recent study of black married couples, Clark-Nicolas and Gray-Little (1991) conclude, "Economic resources [such as economic adequacy, income, education, and occupation] are important predictors of marital quality among low-income groups but are less relevant to middle-income relationships" (p. 645).

Spitze (1991) also notes that although a number of social scientists have discussed an association at the aggregate level between rising divorce rates and increases in female labor force participation, possible linkage processes have only recently begun to be explored, and a direction of causality, if any, has yet to be established. Greenstein

(1990) reports, "There is no consistent positive effect of wives' earnings on marital disruption" (p. 674) and suggests that wives' income may *both* facilitate a decision to leave the marriage *and* stabilize the marriage, lowering the likelihood of disruption. In studies of marital solidarity, "Family assets, rather than husbands' income, significantly predict marital stability" (Piotrkowski et al., 1987, p. 263).

Thus, with regard to role allocations and family outcomes, for many families today, two adults in employed work roles are necessary to ensure stable and sufficient income for meeting household economic needs and fulfilling the family provider role. In spite of increasing rates of labor force participation among even mothers with young children, women continue to be disproportionately involved in family work roles, both in task accomplishment and as managers. Recent research suggests, however, that although role overload is a reality for many dual-earner families—particularly for women—satisfaction and marital quality, and even experiences of role overload, depend somewhat more on spousal preferences and perceptions of fairness than strictly on who does how much of what kind of work. A variety of patterns for balancing employed work and family work have emerged, depending on a number of factors. These include family life cycle stage (Higgins, Duxbury, & Lee, 1994); career commitment and stage; levels of income, assets, and other resources available both within the family and from larger social systems; and individual and family definitions, preferences, competencies, and beliefs.

Family Member Outcomes

Menaghan and Parcel (1991) conclude that research "in the 1980s has well established the existence of role strain in dual-earner households across socioeconomic levels and across household types" (p. 375). The health and mental health consequences of role stress and possible role overload for individual family members are not as well understood. Here, I examine research on family member outcomes according to (a) consequences for mothers, (b) consequences for fathers, and (c) consequences for children.

Consequences for Mothers. Spitze (1991) concludes, "For women, the few differences found in overall levels of life satisfaction and mental health favor the employed [over housewives]" (p. 385). Researchers in one study "found the majority of full-time homemakers dissatisfied with their jobs, with specific negative aspects including . . . monotony, fragmentation, and excessive pace" (p. 385). On the other hand, according to this same study, "The most valued job condition [for housework] was autonomy" (p. 385).

Thompson and Walker (1991) conclude, "Most mothers find looking after small children a predominantly unsettling and irritating experience" (p. 92). At the same time, "Most mothers experience their responsibility for children as both frustrating and a source of meaning." Researchers in one study found

> Rare men who are highly involved with the daily activities of looking after their children experience the same ambivalence about parenthood that mothers have always experienced; they enjoy close, rich, fulfilling relationships with their children, but they also endure frustration, worry, boredom, testiness, and tiredness. (Thompson & Walker, 1991, p. 93)

In other studies, it appears "that both employed and nonemployed wives were less distressed when their husbands did an equal share of the household work" (Menaghan & Parcel, 1991, p. 367). In a review, Moen (1992) concludes,

> The connection between employment and well-being is contingent on a variety of factors in women's lives. Employment may be conducive to greater well-being, but it also can lead to role conflict and overload, especially for mothers of young children....Whether employment leads to beneficial or deleterious outcomes for women who are raising young children seems to depend on a complex calculus of costs and benefits. When the perceived benefits exceed the costs, the overall consequence of employment is salutary. Conversely, when the strains and overloads exceed the rewards, the outcome may be less than positive. (p. 55)

Consequences for Fathers. For fathers, family work has traditionally been connected with the provider role through paid employment, but as Thompson and Walker (1991) point out, "In most families, both women and men are enacting the provider role and contributing earnings to their families" (p. 82). On the other hand, "Men retain responsibility and recognition for provision (p. 82)." Thus, in many families today, wives are seen as "helping" husbands with family provision even when their earnings are crucial for economic viability. Alternatively, "Most mothers, fathers, and researchers continue to see fathers' contributions to parenting as 'helping' but never refer to mothers' contributions in this way" (p. 82).

The consequences of changing family patterns for fathers have only recently begun to be studied. Researchers have found that fathers "are more invested and involved in paid work and marriage than they are in parenthood" (Thompson & Walker, 1991, p. 93). Fathers are often "confused and dissatisfied with their involvement in childrearing"; on the other hand, men "who are more involved with their children feel more competent as parents" (p. 93).

Studies of employment and unemployment show that employment is associated with positive well-being among men. Furthermore, unemployment has "powerful negative effects on [men's] individual well-being" as well as on "the quality of [their] participation in family life" (Menaghan & Parcel, 1991, p. 366). In addition, earned income "enhances self-esteem and a sense of mastery, which in turn increase overall well-being" (p. 366).

Preferences, and satisfaction with the fit between beliefs and reality, seem to be important areas for continuing exploration. For example, researchers have found, "Husbands are most depressed when their wives work against husbands' opposition" (Spitze, 1991, p. 386).

Consequences for Children. Outcomes of changing family patterns for children have been the subject of research studies for a number of years. Belsky (1990) found five "waves" of research since the 1970s. Wave 1—Experimental Day Care—focused on potential deleterious consequences of nonparental care in "high-quality, university-based centers" (p. 893) for children's psychological well-being. Reviewers found "little cause for concern" (p. 893). Subsequent research in Wave 2—Beyond Between-Group Comparisons—was focused on conditions and practices in a variety of child care settings and led to findings that "When group size is large, [staff-child] ratios are poor, and caregivers are untrained or unsupervised, individual attention to children falls victim to the exigencies of coping with an overextended set of resources . . . [and] both quality of care and child well-being are compromised" (p. 894).

For Wave 3—The First Year of Life—recent studies have indicated, "When both quality of care and age of entry into full-time care are taken into account, . . . it is children for whom care of low quality is initiated *in their first year* who function more problematically than all other children" (Belsky, 1990, p. 895). Thus, for some children in some situations, infant day care may constitute a "risk factor." In contrast, a longitudinal study in Sweden found no deleterious correlates of first-year day care experience for children whose mothers "experienced *6 months of paid parental leave* before placing their children in *well-resourced infant day care centers* staffed by *well-trained* and reasonably *well-paid* caregivers" (p. 896).

In Wave 4—Family, Work, and Child Care Contexts—researchers have begun to examine "the complex ecology of human development." This includes not only the quality of nonparental care and the child's age of entry into care but also "family attitudes and processes as well as parents' occupational experiences" (Belsky, 1990, p. 896). According to one study, "Toddlers who develop insecure attachments to both their mothers and their family day-care providers evince the least competence in their play with their peers, but . . . those insecurely attached to their mothers but secure in their relationships with their caregivers function more competently" (p. 897). Thus, cumulative risk and compensatory processes as well as interactions between these factors may be important in understanding outcomes for children.

Finally, in Wave 5—Distinct Ecologies—(which has overlapped with Wave 4), a few recent studies have been "based upon the proposition that developmental processes of influence may actually be distinctly different in the case of children with and without extensive nonparental care experience" (Belsky, 1990, p. 897). For example, one study indicated, "When children begin full-time nonparental care in their first year of life, their later development is predicted by the quality of their day care, but *not* by family factors and processes. Intriguingly, just the reverse is true of children whose full-time care began after their first year" (p. 897). Although much further work needs to be done in this area, Belsky (1990) notes, "To the extent that different processes of development are found to characterize children growing up in contrasting ecologies, this will prove important, not simply for our understanding of the developmental effect of day care, but for general developmental and family theory as well" (p. 898).

Moen (1992) summarizes recent theory and research:

> We know that the key to optimal human development is a stable, predictable environment and that in hectic, unpredictable situations the processes linking children to their care givers begin to deteriorate. . . . Yet the current reality of American society is that the daily life of the child is frequently disjointed, neither stable nor predictable. . . . For many families the mother's salary is essential for the family economy, and her employment is beneficial to her own emotional well-being. At the same time, maternal employment in the context of today's institutional con-

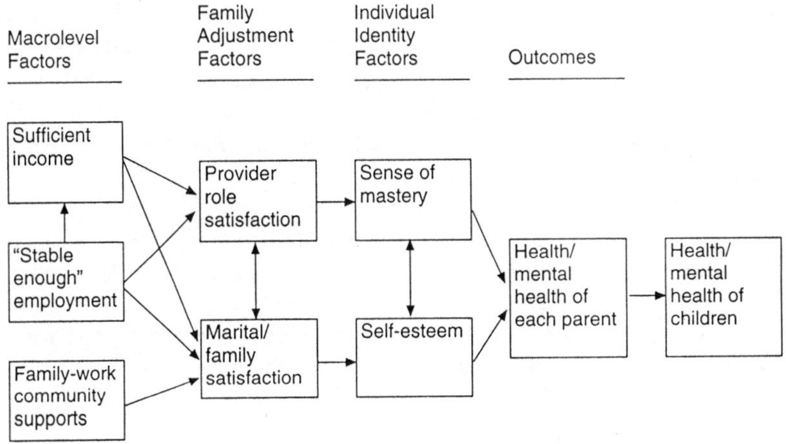

Figure 4.3. Multilevel Factors in Family Member Outcomes

> straints makes family life both more unpredictable and more hectic. We provide no systematic supports for families in the United States, regardless of whether the mother is working; therefore, American families with young children are increasingly placed at risk. (pp. 90-91)

In summary, for individual family members, outcomes of recent changes in family patterns seem to vary between mothers, fathers, and children. Outcomes also appear to be interconnected in a variety of ways with family factors as well as with constraints and opportunities in larger social systems. Figure 4.3 summarizes a number of the factors discussed above. These involve macrolevel, family, and individual factors.

Macrolevel factors include reasonably stable employment for one or both spouses so that family system equilibrium for managing multiple activities and roles can be achieved. Related to this is the need for jobs that provide sufficient income to meet the family's economic needs, including work-related expenses. Particularly when both parents are engaged in employed work, family work supports in the community are of critical importance. These include stable, accessible, affordable, quality child care and youth supervision and care for sick, disabled, or frail elderly family members.

Family adjustment factors involve shared understandings that take into account individual preferences and expectations as well as role assignments that result in satisfaction for each spouse regarding both the provider roles and other family work roles (see Figure 4.1). A variety of patterns of role allocation and shared or gender-based activities are possible. Spouses' satisfaction with both their own and their spouse's role performance in mutually assigned employed work and family work roles are crucial linking factors in understanding outcomes for parents and subsequently for children.

Recent research has identified individual identity factors of sense of mastery and self-esteem as important in understanding health and mental health outcomes for adults. The model in Figure 4.3 suggests that these factors provide links between spouses' family role satisfactions and outcomes for parents. In addition, parents' outcomes are key for understanding children's health and mental health consequences.

STRESSORS AND DIVERSITY

Diversity is an important reality in U.S. society. As Spitze (1991) notes, however, most of the research on families and work "views the middle-class white family as the norm" (p. 382). Social work practitioners and researchers need to continually be attentive to stressors among a variety of types of families.

Some stresses between employed work and family work that need further empirical study are related to the family life cycle. These include role overload for adult children in midlife—particularly women who are caring for frail elderly parents and other members of the kin network (Gerstel & Gallagher, 1993)—and effects of early retirement (Hanks, 1990). Other unique stressors are related to job characteristics and structures, such as shift work (Simon, 1990), women in blue-collar occupations (Kissman, 1990), family businesses (Wicker & Burley, 1991), farm families (Godwin, Draughn, Little, & Marlowe, 1991), and dual-career families (see Schwartz & Scott, 1994; it is estimated that about 7% of couples are "dual-career," p. 300).

Two types of families requiring major focus for understanding particular stresses and overloads are single-adult households with children and families with low-wage earners. I briefly discuss particular kinds of overloads for these two family types.

Single-Parent Households

Although single-parent households face significant risks for role overload and poverty, when adequate income and support are available they can provide a viable and well-functioning social system environment for healthy and satisfied adults and children. Cohen, Johnson, Lewis, and Brook (1990) noted in a recent study, "Both maternal and child problems of psychopathology were elevated in single-mother families. However, these effects were very predominantly accounted for by the low income levels of these families, and where income was adequate no excess risk was apparent" (p. 130).

Moen (1992) notes that by 1988, 19.7% or "one in five families with children present in the United States was maintained by a single-parent mother" (p. 27). Ellwood and Crane (1990) report, "According to several estimates, the majority of children born today will spend some time in a single-parent home" (p. 81).

An examination of Figures 4.1 and 4.2 reveals a number of potential points of stress pileup for a single parent with children. First, unless she—the majority of single parents are women—is able to find and maintain a relatively high-paying job or has substantial child support from her child(ren)'s father, she must essentially juggle three full-time jobs: two jobs to fulfill the provider role plus a full-time family work schedule (see Figure 4.1). In addition, assuming that she is involved in employed work, she will be solely responsible not only for after-hours dependent care, child rearing, and youth supervision but also for arranging all transportation to and from both child care and work, and for any backup care—such as sick care—for both herself and her child(ren) (see Figure 4.2).

With stable employment, sufficient income, and supportive community services (see Figure 4.3), some single parents—both single mothers and single fathers—are able to manage the multiple roles required, find satisfaction in enacting those multiple roles, achieve a sense of mastery and positive self-esteem, and thereby nurture health and well-being for both themselves and their children. Particularly where larger-system economic and community social service supports are not in place, however, dissatisfaction and frustration, lowered self-esteem, depression, and even child abuse can result. These families are at particular risk for family system destabilization in the event of employed work layoff (see Chapter 6), and subsequently for the devastation that can result from chronic poverty (see Chapter 8).

Low-Wage Earner Families

Even in dual-earner families—including extended-family households—more attention must begin to be paid to the macrolevel issues of stable employment, sufficient income, and community supports. For parents in low-wage jobs, child care costs can erode substantially the effort to provide sufficient income through the employed work of both parents. Where employment for either parent is unstable, child care arrangements are likely to be subject to constant change as well. This can result in successive family system transition and reorganization periods and the potential for chronic stress pileup.

KNOWLEDGE GAPS AND FUTURE DIRECTIONS

Although much empirical work has been done, especially recently, in an attempt to better understand families and work, a number of limitations and gaps in knowledge remain to be addressed. As noted above, much more work is needed regarding similarities and differences for diverse types of families in their struggles to balance employed work and family work. For example, possible differences by (a) family structure (e.g., single-parent, remarried, and extended family), (b) class (e.g., high income, middle income, lower-middle income, and low income), and (c) race and ethnicity need to be explored. Research areas need to be examined together rather than isolated in specialized fragments. For example, researchers focusing on employed work and those interested in child care issues could identify important interconnections and interactions. Similarly, knowledge building should expand for understanding interconnections among outcomes for mothers, fathers, and children. Finally, longitudinal studies are critical in understanding change over time and identifying interventions that can make a difference in alleviating stress pileup and role overload. Such understandings will provide a critically needed expanding knowledge base for multilevel work aimed at ensuring better-functioning families and healthy family members.

SOCIAL WORK IMPLICATIONS

The theory and research reviewed in this chapter provides social work practitioners and researchers with empirically based knowledge for elucidating connections across previously arbitrarily drawn lines dividing macro from micro practice. In addition, current knowledge provides workers with a base for normalizing with individuals and families the stress many parents and others are experiencing between employed work and family work. As will be discussed further in Chapter 5, tools for multilevel assessment and evaluation and models for change at multiple system levels are critically needed. With the person-in-environment framework, social workers have vital roles to play in (a) documenting current realities and adding to knowledge, (b) exploring alternatives and choices and developing innovative models for policies and programs, and (c) identifying and examining outcomes of interventions to generate and maintain positive change at multiple systems levels.

SUMMARY

Over the past several decades, average wages in the United States for men have declined. During the same time period, labor force participation by women—particularly mothers with children—has dramatically increased. Many families are now dual-earner households in which both parents are engaged in full-time, year-round employed work. A subset of these families are dual-career couples, in which both partners choose to pursue full-time careers.

Particularly for families with children, there continues to be a full-time family work role, requiring an average of 47 hours of work per week. Women continue to do most of this family work (an average of 33 hours per week, compared with an average of 14 hours per week for men). In addition, mothers are more likely than fathers to fulfill the role of family manager.

When partners are satisfied with employed work arrangements and larger-system environments provide sufficient income, stable employment, and family work community supports—including quality child care—dual-earner families are able to balance employed work and family work, with concomitant healthy outcomes for all family members. For many families with children or other dependents, however—and especially for low-wage earner or single-parent households—role overload from the struggle to fulfill all of the family work roles—manager, provider, decision maker, household maintenance, dependents' care, and child rearing—can result in risk for deleterious health and mental health outcomes for parents and for their children.

Chapter 5

FAMILIES AND WORK
Applications and Tools for Practice

CASE DESCRIPTION

Figures 5.1 and 5.2 provide a genogram and ecomap for the Smith family in 1993; a time line is shown in Figure 3.6 in Chapter 3. Peter (age 24) and Jane (age 23), parents of Kevin (age 3) and Susan (age 1), have been referred to an Employee Assistance Program (EAP) worker, Marvin, by Peter's union representative. Officials at the auto plant where Peter has worked for the past 5 years have announced that it will be closing in 6 months. Peter's friends at work noticed that following the announcement, Peter several times came to work drunk. Jane, who works part-time at the union hall while her mother watches the two children, encouraged Peter to heed his friends' advice to see a counselor, noting that they have been fighting more since the plant closing announcement and that she would like to "talk to someone about our family arguments and tensions with the kids." Peter reluctantly agreed to go with Jane to see a "family counselor."

Currently, Peter works full-time at the auto assembly plant. Based on Peter's union wages and Jane's income from her part-time job at the union hall, the Smiths recently began buying a small home in the city, with an adjustable-rate mortgage. They are able to meet monthly expenses, but have no savings for an emergency.

Peter has made many friends at work. Since their move into the city, Jane has seen less of her friends from high school who live in the suburbs, but she has begun to make friends at the union hall.

Some of the arguments between Peter and Jane have resulted from Jane's requests that Peter "take more responsibility" in the home, now that there are two young children to care for and she has a part-time job. Peter's father worked for years at the same auto assembly plant where Peter now

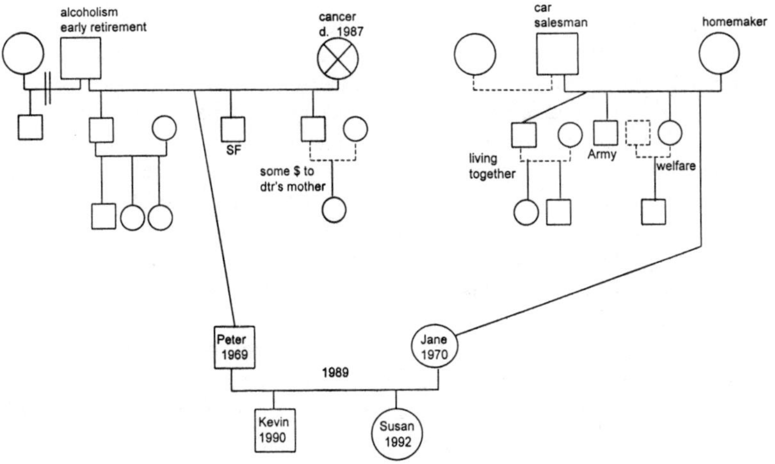

Figure 5.1. 1993 Smith Family Genogram

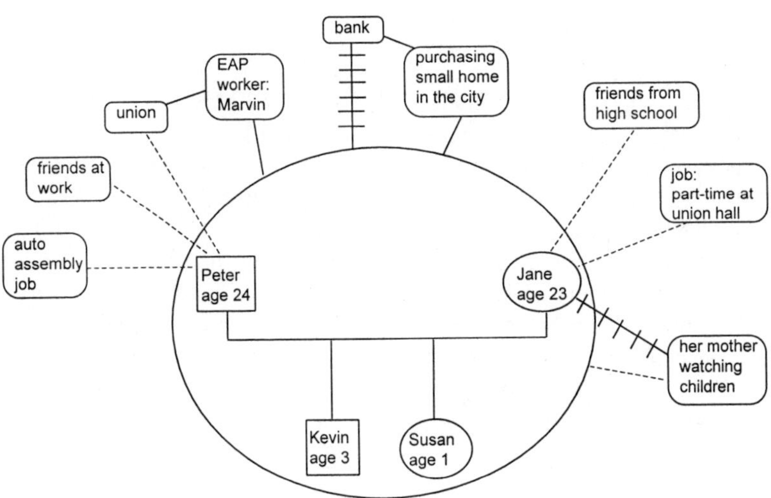

Figure 5.2. 1993 Smith Family Ecomap

works. The father recently took early retirement. He has had problems with alcoholism for many years. His wife, who died 5 years ago of cancer, was a homemaker; and Peter expects Jane to play the same role as his mother. He has very ambivalent feelings about Jane's working outside the home, even part-time, but he admits that they might not have been able to purchase a home of their own without her income.

An additional complication is that Jane's mother, who has been looking after the two young grandchildren—Kevin and Susan—free of charge, recently informed Jane that she plans to look for employment now that all of her own children are launched. Consequently, Jane must find child care for Kevin and Susan if she plans to continue in paid employment.

In this chapter, I discuss work with and on behalf of families experiencing the normative stress of struggling to balance employed work and family work in the context of the current U.S. social system. First, I present tools for assessment designed to assist practitioners and researchers in understanding the family in context. Next, I discuss interventions and evaluation of change at various social systems levels. Finally, I delineate strategies for development and change in larger social systems, including advocacy, empowerment, and knowledge and consensus building.

TOOLS FOR FAMILY ASSESSMENT

General tools for family assessment have been discussed in Chapter 3. Here, I assume that the practitioner or researcher has established, through a more general assessment of the family, that at least one family member is experiencing some kind of role strain or role overload in balancing work and family tasks. The discussion of general family tools such as the ecomap, genogram, and time line, as well as exploration of expenses and resources, is focused on issues regarding employed work and family work. In addition, I present a guide for discussing household time and tasks management.

Family Budget

To work effectively with families experiencing work-family overloads, social workers and other human service professionals must have a clear understanding of financial realities in the family. Figure 5.3 provides an instrument for detailed discussion of a family's weekly or

INCOME:					
Net pay (after taxes & deductions):	his	$			
	hers	$			
Other		$			
Total Income:				$	
EXPENDITURES:					
Fixed:					
Mortgage or rent		$			
Property taxes		$			
Other taxes (e.g., income and social security taxes not withheld by employer)		$			
Alimony, child support		$			
Day care		$			
Installment and credit card payments		$			
Insurance (auto, life, health, other)		$			
Savings and investments (emergency fund, investment fund, vacation fund, education fund, other)		$			
Subtotal, fixed:			$		
Variable:					
Food		$			
Other grocery items (e.g., soap, laundry detergent, diapers, pet food, etc.)		$			
Utilities:	gas/oil	$			
	electricity	$			
	water/sewer	$			
Telephone		$			
Home maintenance		$			
Furnishings		$			
Home improvement		$			
Automobile:	gas and oil	$			
	routine maintenance	$			
	repairs	$			
Public transportation		$			
Clothing:	hers	$			
	his	$			
	child(ren)	$			
Laundry and dry cleaning		$			
Personal care (e.g., haircuts, gym or fitness membership, etc.)		$			
Medical, dental, and pharmacy bills not covered by insurance		$			
Educational expenses		$			
Personal money or allowance (including lunch money):	hers	$			
	his	$			
	child(ren)	$			
Entertainment, recreation, gifts		$			
Contributions		$			
Miscellaneous		$			
Subtotal, variable:			$		
Total Expenses:				$	
TOTAL INCOME - TOTAL EXPENSES:				(+)	$
			or	(-)	$

Week or Month: ______________________

Figure 5.3. Family Budget (Weekly or Monthly)

monthly income and expenditure flows. Data from this household budget provides both the practitioner and family members—such as

Peter and Jane—with a clearer picture of (a) whether income is sufficient to cover normal expenses, (b) whether there are areas of unusual expenditures that are temporarily putting stress on household finances, and (c) whether various family members are satisfied with current income and expenditure patterns or would prefer to see changes in one or more aspects of income provision or outlays. Discussion of "other" income may signal the extent to which the family has access to social support from one or more asset pools, such as savings, property, or extended-family gifts or loans (Sherraden, 1991).

Discussion with the family of income and expenditures should take place during the assessment phase. This information can then be utilized by the practitioner and family members in short-term planning for coping if there is an immediate financial or other family crisis. It can also be used in longer-term planning around possible shifts in income streams, for example, a family member entering or reentering employment, job search activities for obtaining a higher-paying job, or training for upgrading skills, as well as in expenditures such as searching for affordable child care, locating affordable housing, dealing with debts, education in how to use and manage credit, and effective budgeting and management of limited income. See Figure 7.1 in Chapter 7 for a summary of Peter and Jane Smith's family budget 2 years after the plant closing.

Employed Work-Family Work Ecomap

As delineated in Figure 4.2, an ecomap of current family roles and extrafamily role relationships can elicit discussion of stressors as well as social resources and supports at community and larger-system levels. Current arrangements for full-time versus part-time employment, nonparental child care and supervision, sick care, and care of other dependent family members must be explored to understand various aspects of role allocation and sources of potential role overload for one or more family members. Current and past stability versus instability in these three system levels (family, community, and larger systems) may provide clues for better understanding current stress pileup. See Figure 5.2, for example, for an ecomap of the Smith family at the time of the plant closing in 1993.

Supports and tensions created within and by the employed-work environment need to be understood. For example, how flexible are employers and to what extent does the employment environment accommodate family needs such as parental leave following birth (or adoption) or taking time off to care for a sick child? Extent of support from extended-family members and friends and quality and accessibility of nonparental child care and supervision are other important areas for exploration and understanding.

The family's life cycle stage is another important area for examination. Exploration should include spouses' commitment to particular jobs and to building a career; responsibilities for care of an infant, for one or more frail elderly parents, or for a disabled family member; and safety for and ability of children and youth to participate in household maintenance and self-care activities.

Household Time and Tasks Management

Figure 5.4 provides practitioners and family members with a guide to discussion of the various family work roles. These include the manager subrole, tasks involved in each aspect of family work, and time spent performing tasks. A number of activities and roles are essential to ensure that the family social system functions as an effective organizational unit. These role arenas include (a) the provider role(s), (b) household maintenance, (c) family decision making and communication, (d) dependents' care, and (e) children and youth supervision and socialization.

In a family interview during the assessment phase, a worker might assist family members with filling in the information in Figure 5.4. Alternatively, the family might be asked to take the form home to fill it out and bring the completed form to a subsequent session. Discussion of the roles and tasks—and the time and energy commitments necessary for successful role performance—can help practitioners, researchers, and family members to see, perhaps for the first time, previously invisible aspects of family life and family work. Because many of these rather common and ordinary tasks are performed routinely in millions of households throughout society, the knowledge and skills required for successful accomplishment have often been ignored. In previous times, girls and young women often were expected to learn homemaking skills in their families of origin and to enact their family work roles unquestioningly for their husbands and children. Now, however, structural economic changes discussed in Chapter 4 require increasing numbers of wives and mothers to participate in employed work and the provider role. In addition, more positive attitudes have emerged toward women who combine careers and family work.

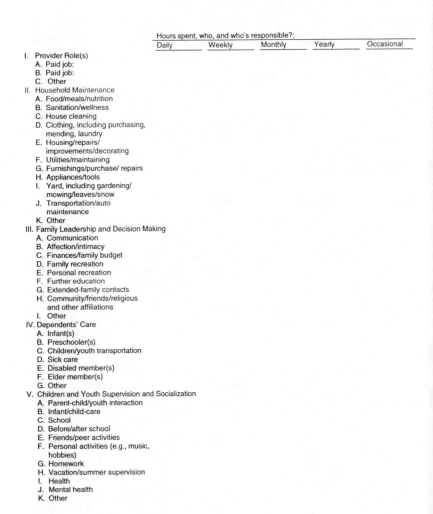

	Hours spent, who, and who's responsible?:				
	Daily	Weekly	Monthly	Yearly	Occasional
I. Provider Role(s)					
A. Paid job:					
B. Paid job:					
C. Other					
II. Household Maintenance					
A. Food/meals/nutrition					
B. Sanitation/wellness					
C. House cleaning					
D. Clothing, including purchasing, mending, laundry					
E. Housing/repairs/ improvements/decorating					
F. Utilities/maintaining					
G. Furnishings/purchase/ repairs					
H. Appliances/tools					
I. Yard, including gardening/ mowing/leaves/snow					
J. Transportation/auto maintenance					
K. Other					
III. Family Leadership and Decision Making					
A. Communication					
B. Affection/intimacy					
C. Finances/family budget					
D. Family recreation					
E. Personal recreation					
F. Further education					
G. Extended-family contacts					
H. Community/friends/religious and other affiliations					
I. Other					
IV. Dependents' Care					
A. Infant(s)					
B. Preschooler(s)					
C. Children/youth transportation					
D. Sick care					
E. Disabled member(s)					
F. Elder member(s)					
G. Other					
V. Children and Youth Supervision and Socialization					
A. Parent-child/youth interaction					
B. Infant/child-care					
C. School					
D. Before/after school					
E. Friends/peer activities					
F. Personal activities (e.g., music, hobbies)					
G. Homework					
H. Vacation/summer supervision					
I. Health					
J. Mental health					
K. Other					

Figure 5.4. Household Time and Tasks Management

Making visible for both families and society the necessary components—management skills, time, and energy for accomplishment of tasks—for successful family work becomes critical for addressing role allocation issues and role overloads. Figure 7.2 in Chapter 7 provides a time and tasks picture of the Smith family 2 years after the plant closing—and after extensive work with Marvin, their EAP worker.

Family Genogram and Work

Construction of a family genogram as delineated in general in Chapter 3 can enable discussion of beliefs and patterns of employed work and family work in the current household as well as in the families of origin of the partners. As indicated in Chapter 4 (see Figure 4.1), beliefs, preferences, expectations, and explicit or implicit family rules shape the family's working model of how activities are allocated to ensure system equilibrium in family work roles. Figure 5.1 shows a genogram of Peter and Jane's extended family at the time of the plant closing.

Particularly where the current working model is very different from the roles, definitions, beliefs, and rules learned in one or both families of origin, criticism from extended-family members can cause stress in the household even if both spouses agree that the current equilibrium is necessary. On the other hand, for some couples, constant and seemingly unresolvable conflict over roles and rules may be the only working model discernible, resulting in chronic arguing, tension and bitterness, marital dissatisfaction and instability, and even marital dissolution.

The struggle to balance employed work and family work involves both the family and larger system constraints and supports. Discussion of the various system-level factors indicated in Figure 4.3 in Chapter 6 can assist practitioners and family members—including extended-family members where appropriate—to perceive and assess issues causing stress that may result in deleterious health or mental health outcomes for parents and children. Exploration and assessment of not only macrolevel factors—sufficient income, "stable-enough" employment, and family work community supports—but also family and individual factors—including satisfaction with the provider and other family roles, and each spouse's self-esteem and sense of mastery—can lead to identification of areas of tension and stress as well as possible change points for examination or negotiation.

Family Time Line and Work

Delineation of a family's history and chronology can elicit discussion of career aspirations, employment histories, financial and provider role expectations and changes, and family life cycle patterns. Where changes have been forced by external systems, discussion of larger-system realities may provide a common path to mutual understanding. This might include a lessening of spouses blaming each other for dissatisfaction and frustration. (For a time line of the Smith family at the time of the plant closing, see Figure 3.6 in Chapter 3.)

Exploration of Community Resources

Discussion with the family of what they know of community resources and constraints can enable assessment of current employment and employer practices; family social services and public policies at local, state, and national levels; and the family's access to available resources. Barriers to services should be explored with the family. These might include lack of reliable transportation and affordable high-quality child care and youth supervision as well as gaps in policies and services in particular neighborhoods or areas, for example, in some inner cities or rural counties. Marvin, Peter and Jane's EAP worker, will need to assess not only strengths and stressors for the Smith family but also resources and resource gaps in the neighborhood and local community—which are related to state and national policies and programs, as well as to global socioeconomic change.

In summary, use of a variety of assessment tools that focus on roles and role overloads in today's families can enable practitioners, researchers, and families to better understand this previously invisible and now normative stressor in U.S. society. The purpose of such an assessment is knowledge that results in planning and implementation of interventions and multilevel change. The ultimate goal is to enable currently overloaded and overstressed families successfully to balance employed work and family work roles and ensure healthy families and family members and well-functioning larger social systems.

MULTILEVEL INTERVENTIONS AND EVALUATION

Interventions with and on behalf of clients at multiple systems levels are likely to be necessary for effective work in preventing and relieving employed work-family work role overloads. Two types of interventions operate at the family system level: (a) family life education, and (b) clinical social work with individuals and families. In addition, I discuss development in larger systems, including needed changes at

(c) neighborhood and local, (d) state and national, and (e) global social system levels.

Family Life Education

As employed work becomes by necessity a more salient life role for most women—as it has traditionally been for men (Pottick, 1989)—there is a need for preventive family life education that addresses family attitudes, preferences, and beliefs about roles and how to combine employed work and family work. Studies of college students have found that men and women are equally committed to careers, and that they are similar in viewing family life as important (Covin & Brush, 1991); differences have been found in how women and men students view employed work-family work trade-offs (DiBenedetto & Tittle, 1990). Areas that need further discussion and research are the issue of combining employed work—particularly when it is regarded as a career—and family work, as well as varieties of workable solutions to role overload for both men and women.

Particularly for families negotiating more gender equality in parenting responsibilities, parent education that directly involves both mothers and fathers—such as Jane and Peter—should explicitly address fathers' needs (Meyers, 1993). Curriculum content should foster parents' "knowledge about care-giving" (p. 450) as well as skills in "marital communication" and "child communication" (p. 451). Although programs that address these knowledge and skill content areas are likely to be useful for both men and women, family life education has often focused primarily on work with mothers. This focus reinforces traditional gendered role structures. In a changing social context, basic underlying assumptions for both practitioners and agencies must be examined and appropriate changes must be made in practice and programming.

Clinical Social Work

Clinical work with stressed families should be focused where possible on involving *both* partners, because role overload in today's families is usually not a one-person problem. "Normalizing" the overload to reduce anxiety for family members may be necessary prior to a careful examination of current roles, use of resources, organizational structures in the family, beliefs and preferences, and specific sources of stress as well as family strengths and previous coping strategies.

For some families, assistance with identifying, accessing, and managing additional outside resources—such as stable nonparental child care or household help—may enable the family to resume normal functioning. Of course, this intervention strategy assumes that adequate and affordable child care and other services are available in the neighborhood or local community. Where services are in place, some family members may need knowledge of or help in developing skills in accessing service systems. In addition, the family may need to learn skills in effective management of ongoing relationships with caregivers or other service staff.

Another group of families may need help with budgeting or decisions regarding family lifestyles relative to who works how many hours to provide for family needs. For some families, deciding to cut back on certain expenditures may enable one or both parents to balance employed work and family work roles better.

For other families—such as the Smiths—help may be needed in finding more stable employment or in setting longer-term goals for further education and higher income levels. Again, such strategies are dependent on employment, wage, and education structures in larger social systems.

Other families may need assistance in establishing new communication and negotiation patterns and perhaps in restructuring employed work-family work roles, beliefs, and rules. As Brett and Yogev (1988) indicate, this restructuring is likely to involve consideration of (a) his employed work; (b) his family work; (c) her employed work; (d) her family work; and (e) couple factors such as family life cycle stage, number of children, access to paid help, and the family's financial power (p. 160). Helping family members change their personal roles and their shared family internal working model to achieve a new family system equilibrium may involve difficult and emotion-charged clinical work. Change may be particularly difficult where belief systems have been adopted unexamined from one or both families of origin. Such work may be necessary, however, for satisfaction, self-esteem, and a sense of mastery to improve for one or both spouses.

Another new area for discussion of personal and family change may be the interface between family and jobs. Swiss and Walker (1993) delineate "A Call to Action" (p. 228) for family members to make their voices heard collectively in regard to changes in the employed-work environment as well as in federal legislation. Empowering clients in *family* systems has been a traditional area for professional discussion;

empowerment of clients within *larger* systems is a relatively new area for dialogue, knowledge and skills development, and action.

In all of these areas—resource management, role restructuring, and empowerment—families will be helped not only by direct clinical work but by participation in ongoing evaluation of what works for them. In collaboration with agency practitioners and researchers, client family members can assist in identifying resources and resource gaps in neighborhood and local community systems. Gaps may include quality and affordability of nonparental child care, elder and disabled care, and sick care. Accessibility of services and transportation needs can also be assessed, and the extent of difficulties can be tracked across agency caseloads.

In addition, families can provide data regarding employment stability, wage levels, and adequacy of employment benefits, as well as employers' flexibility in assisting family members to balance family and employee responsibilities. Family members might also participate in community development and social change efforts, providing data on both positive and negative impacts of organizational and governmental policies and programs.

Where appropriate, family members and practitioners in collaboration can track role restructuring and other important shifts in the family. They might also participate in research that provides data on changes in levels of individual family members' job and marital and family satisfaction; self-esteem; sense of mastery; and health and mental health.

Families can also become partners with agencies in program evaluation, such as by making suggestions and providing feedback on family life education programs and clinical and other agency services. For all of these evaluation and research areas, usable, valid, and reliable measures as well as interview or other data-collection protocols will need to be identified or developed. This should be done in collaboration with and with feedback from practitioners and client family members. Common measures and procedures will enable sharing of data and comparison of studies across families, agencies and organizations, neighborhoods, local communities, states, and even nations.

Thus, evaluation of clinical services becomes a multifaceted enterprise that can take on numerous forms. These might include documentation, tracking of needs and resources, before and after or single-system design studies (which, with clients' permission, can be pooled into more formal research studies), and formal evaluations of particular programs and services based on practitioners', clients', and agencies' needs and interests.

Neighborhood and Local Community Development

As is evident in the description of the Smith family and the discussion of clinical work with families, the presence or absence of social system support components in the family's neighborhood and local community are key to effective interventions for healthy functioning of the family as a system and of individual members. Here, I discuss the following key support components: (a) economic structures, (b) political planning and support, and (c) cultural values and belief systems.

Economic Structures. For family members to effectively fulfill provider roles in the family system, there must be opportunities available for employment or self-employment in the "walking" neighborhood, or if the jobs are outside the immediate neighborhood in the larger local community, reliable transportation to and from employment must be available and accessible.

In addition, employment must be compensated by wages that enable family members to provide the goods and services needed in the family household. Alternatively, in social systems in which citizens are not willing to ensure minimum wage levels for family provision, there will be a need to subsidize—on a stable ongoing basis—essential goods and services. Subsidies may need to include food, housing, utilities, transportation, health care, education, child care, before- and after-school care, sick care, youth activities, frail elder care, and disabled care.

It is essential that social workers such as Marvin know the neighborhoods in which client families live. Home visits and walking tours of neighborhoods can provide practitioners and researchers with a rich understanding of community supports and economic and other barriers. A bus trip with a family member can provide a clearer understanding of the time involved for a working mother to get to and from a job, child care, grocery shopping, banking, shopping for clothing and supplies (e.g., school supplies), laundromats, social service agencies, and so forth. Based on these and other data, social work agencies must begin to take leading roles in developing economic and family supports in neighborhoods and communities to ensure stable provider as well as family work environments for healthy family functioning.

Political Planning and Support. Increasingly, to work effectively with stressed families and ensure stable household economic provision, practitioners and agencies must expand their collaboration with governmental personnel to address such areas as neighborhood planning; economic development; stable and adequate wages or subsidy mechanisms; and affordable, accessible, high-quality social services for all citizens. In some countries in the world, home ownership seems to have been a key factor in stabilizing the lives of families over the past several decades (see, e.g., Blake, 1991).

As discussed above, practitioners and researchers—and, where appropriate, client family members—can play key roles in documenting both positive and negative impacts of a variety of neighborhood and local community efforts. They also can participate in supporting and working for long-term development and change. Social service agencies can play important roles in catalyzing discussion, negotiation, and action planning among a variety of actors in the public, private, and nonprofit sectors. The goals are both understanding how stress from larger systems impacts family systems and developing supportive structures and programs to ensure healthy communities, neighborhoods, and families.

Cultural Values and Belief Systems. Social work practitioners—such as Marvin—who embody professional values of social and economic justice, self-determination, and respect for diversity can become key players in the development of shared neighborhood and community beliefs and values. Shared working models should foster choices for a diversity of peoples, access to opportunities, and participation in the responsibility of developing community and neighborhood social systems that support healthy families.

State and National Development

Where entrenched elite local political structures exclude groups of citizens and block development and change efforts, it becomes necessary for organizations and structures in larger social systems—for example, at the state and national levels—to establish regulations and programs to equalize social benefits and opportunities for all citizens. It can also be argued that because of radical changes in transportation and communication systems—as well as the development of private corporations that cross local, state, and even national boundaries—

states are increasingly simply subsystems in the larger national socio-economic, sociopolitical, sociocultural system that is the United States of America (see Figure 2.3). The question then becomes not, "Shall we as U.S. citizens create or *not* create state and national social systems?" but instead, "What *kind* of social systems will we develop?"

Assuming that to ensure healthy future social systems, children must be raised and educated to become healthy and contributing adults, the value of supporting families in their various family work roles seems self-evident. Within this working model of assumptions and beliefs, a variety of rules, roles, and structural arrangements can be debated, decided on, tried out, evaluated, and changed where necessary.

For example, there seems to be some consensus in the United States that universal access to health care is needed. The structural form that this access might take, however, is open to debate, legislative decision making, and ongoing evaluation and change. Similarly, social workers and other human service professionals—including EAP workers like Marvin—must be involved at state and national levels in debates and decisions regarding full employment and minimum wage levels; housing (including home ownership) and utilities subsidies; education (including continuing education and training in a changing economy); and employer responsiveness to such issues as parental leave, temporary versus part-time versus full-time employment, on-site child care, time off to care for ill or disabled family members, flextime arrangements, and other "family policy" issues (see Chilman, 1988a, 1988b; Googins, 1991; Hartman, 1993; Kamerman, 1986; Moen, 1992; Voydanoff, 1987; Zimmerman, 1988). This involvement might include work as individual citizens or professionals, through professional organizations, and through agency (e.g., union) participation in collaborative projects and coalitions.

State and national private, nonprofit, and public financing mechanisms, including taxation systems, must be analyzed and evaluated to determine positive as well as negative impacts on the healthy functioning of local communities, neighborhoods, and families. Where deleterious consequences are documented, mechanisms need to be changed. What kinds of policies and programs are most effective at which systems levels should be subject to debate and ongoing evaluation and development. Practitioners, researchers, and client family members all need to see themselves, as citizens, as participants in various roles at a variety of social systems levels. (For discussion of professional policy practice knowledge and skills, see Jansson, 1994.)

Global Changes

It is clear that understanding—let alone evaluating and changing—the global socioeconomic system is a daunting undertaking. On the other hand, it also clear that with increasing economic interdependence and new technologies making possible instantaneous and ongoing communication, exchange, and decision making across the planet, the question is again not "whether" but "what kind" of social systems we as citizens of Planet Earth will decide to develop. Alternatively, if we fail to participate, someone else will decide for us. Thus, such issues as global economic development; whether and how to manage global markets; and the impact of economic changes on component social systems of nations, communities, and families become relevant topics for social work knowledge building and practice.

Recent research makes clear that in addressing family and employment role overload issues, interventions and changes are needed not only at individual and family levels but also at neighborhood, local, state, and even national and international levels. Because of diversity in family structures, cultural backgrounds and beliefs, and life cycle stages, it is likely that no single policy or program will meet the resource and support needs of every family. Strategies are needed to enable ongoing development of coordinated policies and programs at various systems levels, based on input, feedback, and other kinds of participation from both professionals and clients.

STRATEGIES FOR SOCIAL CHANGE

To ensure multilevel development and effective participation in needed changes in larger social systems, a number of different strategies—which can be utilized separately or in combinations—are available to social work practitioners and other human service professionals. I discuss three types of strategies here: (a) advocacy, (b) empowerment, and (c) building knowledge for consensus.

Advocacy

Advocacy has been and continues to be a traditional social work method for change efforts at multiple systems levels. It includes case advocacy and class advocacy (Jansson, 1994). *Case advocacy* to address issues of employment and family role overloads might involve a practitioner intervening on behalf of a particular family to obtain such resources as nonparental child care or before- and after-school care. *Class advocacy* might involve social workers negotiating with employers or existing agencies to expand resources available in the community. Such resources might include child care, parental leave, flextime in employment hours, or governmental child care subsidies.

Often, class advocacy is an important strategy for development of neighborhood and local resources through policies and programs at state and national levels. A local employer may argue that a decision by the company to provide "extra" benefits for all employees—such as day care or parental leave—would escalate labor costs and put the company at a competitive disadvantage relative to other corporations. If such policies and programs are mandated for *all* companies in the state or nation, then the competitive advantage in *not* providing such programs would evaporate.

Advocacy can assume a conflict mode of operation, in which the advocate(s) confront(s) agency staff, governmental bureaucrats, employers, legislators, and other social systems actors and decision makers to pressure them to make available resources to which a client family is entitled or to develop needed resources for clients who are currently unserved or underserved. Case advocacy is usually seen as a strategy that expert professionals do on behalf of client families, especially when families do not have the knowledge, time, or energy to participate as citizens in the intervention efforts. Within the profession, advocacy —particularly class advocacy—is often seen as a specialized practice area for a relatively small number of "macro"—even "radical"—practitioners who may have to be willing to work in unstable employment settings, outside established agencies and structures, and for low to very low pay (change makers often have very low status and little power to negotiate a high wage).

Empowerment

Related to advocacy but with a somewhat different focus and emphasis, an empowerment strategy to achieve change in larger social systems involves clients and others as citizens *in* the change process (Graber et al., in press; Jansson, 1994). For groups of neighborhood families, each overloaded with employed work and family work responsibilities and dilemmas, an empowerment strategy may be to (a) assist them as a group in putting together networks of resources for support and mutual problem solving, (b) enlist their help in documenting needs and gaps in services, (c) teach family members how to work existing resource systems and then perhaps teach them how to teach these skills to their neighbors, and (d) organize opportunities for clients to interact with decision makers to advocate on their own behalf.

The goal of an empowerment strategy, from a professional perspective, is that families will move from being clients needing services to becoming citizens involved in ongoing development of social systems that support and enable healthy families and family members. Thus, at the neighborhood level, as a part of receiving services, families can be asked to identify ways in which they might subsequently participate in helping other neighbors in need (Graber et al., in press). At the local level, family members might be asked to participate in planning and implementing a variety of programs and services (Graber et al., in press). Such services might require policy and program support and change at state and national levels as well (Vosler & Nair, 1993; Vosler & Ozawa, 1992).

An empowerment strategy might also include enabling family members to identify and lobby legislators. In addition, it might more generally encourage participation in analysis of proposed policies and in all aspects of the political process—including community organizations, political parties, and social groups and movements. At each of these levels, using an empowerment strategy, practitioners work alongside family members as fellow citizens in development efforts that affect both clients and professionals—each of whom is both participant and actor in a variety of social systems.

Knowledge Building and Consensus

A third strategy for social development and social change in larger systems involves building a rigorous empirical knowledge base that can be utilized for consensus-based interventions—including shifts in cultural belief systems at multiple systems levels. This strategy involves documentation, evaluation, and basic research using a variety of social science methods and models. The goal is to develop a continuously expanding knowledge base for social work practice. Such knowledge is critical for understanding current systems functioning as well as resource gaps and, in the future, development of effective policies and programs that address the employed work-family work role overload dilemma.

As Googins (1991) points out, conflicts occur and changes may be needed for (a) individuals, (b) families, (c) workplaces, and (d) society as a whole (p. 19). Voydanoff (1988, p. 16) notes that research studies are needed to document effects of "family-oriented personnel policies" for individuals and families. Zimmerman (1992) discusses the need for "a consensus . . . that will allow governments to be more helpful to individuals and families, and thereby change the present course of government policy" (p. 166). Adding to the complexity, Moen (1992) argues for a "'life-course' solution" that takes into account various family life cycle stages, creating "more options and a greater diversity for both men and women in youth, early adulthood, mid-life, and the later years" (p. 129).

Knowledge building regarding effective policies and programs for supporting families in employed work and family work should include reviews of arrangements in other countries. (See, for example, Blake & Lam, 1993; Hewlett, Ilchman, & Sweeney, 1986; Kalleberg & Rosenfeld, 1990; Leira, 1992; Marlow, 1991; Moen, 1989.) In the United States, the relative effectiveness of public versus private sector alternatives—in what combinations and at which systems levels—needs review and analysis (Meyers, 1990). For example, some studies of employment-based programs have begun to emerge (Christensen & Staines, 1990; Galinsky & Stein, 1990; Goff, Mount, & Jamison, 1990; Swiss & Walker, 1993), but this research area is in need of significant expansion both theoretically and empirically (Raabe, 1990; see also Lambert, 1993).

There is a critical need for knowledge development and ongoing evaluation and research in such specific areas as flextime, on-site day care centers, flexible use of vacation time (e.g., for sick care, doctor's or school appointments, etc.), school-based before- and after-school care, community-based day care (including before- and after-school and school vacation care), a variety of lengths of parental leave (perhaps in combination with a return to part-time work), various kinds of job security experiments for one or both parents, part-time versus full-time work, work-at-home employment, and diverse ways of financing such arrangements—including private sector service provision or subsidy, public sector service provision or subsidy, and combinations of these.

Various services and funding mechanisms are being studied in the United States and in other nations (see, e.g., Kamerman, 1986; Leira, 1992; Marlow, 1991; Moen, 1989). Interdisciplinary work in this area is critical and should involve social science research that includes social workers, sociologists and anthropologists, psychologists, economists, and political scientists. Direct service practitioners are often the first to notice resource gaps as well as negative impacts of new programs and policies. In collaboration with individual clients and families, they can document both problems and effective interventions. There is a need for the development of common evaluation tools and measures for various levels, including individual (e.g., self-esteem, sense of mastery, depression, physical health); family (satisfaction with roles, conflict, healthy functioning, economic strain, time and tasks stress, etc.); and social health indicators at neighborhood, local, state, and national levels. A variety of national data sets are needed for comparisons between and across nations.

Based on and contributing to this ongoing knowledge building, social work practitioners and researchers can participate by (a) documenting individual and family change, (b) evaluating programs that demonstrate short- and long-term gains toward healthier families, neighborhoods, and local communities, and (c) documenting negative and positive impacts of policies made at state and national levels on individuals, families, and communities. Based on the best information available, choices can be made and then evaluated for consequences. Programs that work can be publicized and replicated when appropriate. A variety of actors—including Marvin and the Smith family—at multiple systems levels must share in making changes, evaluating those changes for all citizens, and continuing to develop effective social systems that support and enhance life for a diversity of families and family members.

SUMMARY

Social work with families struggling with the normative stress of balancing employed work and family work requires tools for family assessment that focus both on the family and on larger social systems. Assessment tools include the family budget, employed work and family work ecomaps, understanding of household time and task management, the family genogram, the family time line, and exploration of community resources. Multilevel interventions must not only focus on the family system—using currently available family life education and clinical social work methods—but also address resources and resource gaps in larger systems, including methods for neighborhood and local community development, state and national policy and program innovation, and attention to global socioeconomic changes. Strategies for change in larger social systems can involve case and class advocacy, empowerment, and knowledge and consensus building.

Chapter 6

FAMILIES AND UNEMPLOYMENT
Theory and Research

In this chapter, I review current social science research and theory regarding a potentially catastrophic family stressor event: one (or more) of the family's providers becoming unemployed. I begin the chapter with a brief historical overview of the development of unemployment theory and research. I delineate current theories and theoretical frameworks, including key concepts for understanding unemployment in family systems. A review of research findings follows. This includes attention to particular vulnerabilities related to unemployment for older workers, women, minorities, and persons with less education. Finally, I summarize knowledge gaps and future directions for knowledge building and discuss implications for social work practice.

HISTORY OF THEORY AND RESEARCH

Social science knowledge building in the United States with regard to the impact of unemployment on workers and their families can be divided into four very general phases. The first phase consisted of studies in the 1930s of primarily working-class unemployed workers and their families during the Great Depression. During the 1970s, two additional types of studies emerged: community-level correlation studies and studies of health consequences of unemployment for individual workers. During the 1980s, U.S. workers experienced increasing unemployment as a result of plant closings. This provided researchers with the opportunity to examine the direction of proposed causal links between unemployment and health—as well as mental health—outcomes. More recently, unemployment studies have diversified in a variety of directions, using different methods of study. These efforts include international comparisons, the use of nationally representative U.S. data sets, and examination of stressors and supportive resources at multiple social systems levels. Some of these studies involve diverse types of individual workers, the worker's family as a whole or other family members, and the roles of the community and structures in more macro social systems—such as local, state, and national employment and unemployment programs and policies.

Depression Era Studies

During the Great Depression in the 1930s, pioneering social science researchers studied the impact of unemployment on primarily working-class individual workers as well as other family members, including wives, young children, and adolescents. Bakke (1940a, 1940b) used a number of methods, including (a) 200 interviews with a random sample of 2,000 families in New Haven, Connecticut (in 1933); (b) small, intensive case studies (from 1932 to 1939); and (c) interviews with service providers. He documented threats to unemployed men's sense of economic security and self-reliance as well as changes in their roles and social relationships.

Komarovsky (1940) interviewed 59 families in New York City (in 1935 and 1936) in which the male head of the family had been unemployed for at least one year. She found (a) changes in family roles as some wives and adolescents, for financial reasons, had to move into employment; (b) threats to the status and authority of the former worker in his relationships with his wife and children; and (c) self-blame and social isolation for some workers and other family members.

In a 1940 study of 180 New York City families on Home Relief or Works Progress Administration (WPA) programs, Ginzberg (1943) found that especially for older men, the Great Depression had depleted their savings and left them with little hope for reemployment. Follow-up interviews in 1941 and 1942 revealed that as a result of U.S. economic shifts in preparation for World War II, a majority of these discouraged workers were reemployed and off relief programs (p. 170). Two other studies during these years—one using data from University of Michigan sociology students (Angell, 1936) and the other based on data from a clinical sample of families at the Institute for Juvenile Research in Chicago (Cavan & Ranck, 1938)—produced findings that some families coped well with the crisis of the Great Depression and others did not cope well at all.

Throughout the 1930s, the Institute of Human Development at the University of California, Berkeley, annually collected data on children and their families in two longitudinal studies: the Oakland Growth Study (167 children and their families) and the Berkeley Guidance Study (214 children and their families) (Elder & Rockwell, 1985, p. 44). These data were later used to study long-term effects of unemployment and hardship on families and grown-up children (Elder, 1974).

Unemployment Studies in the 1970s

Two very different types of unemployment research emerged in the 1970s. Brenner (1973), in *Mental Illness and the Economy,* using New York state data, demonstrated a negative association between employment indices and rates of hospitalization for mental illness. Although these findings cannot be generalized from aggregate community-level rates to individual workers and their families (Dooley & Catalano, 1988), Brenner's research led to a variety of subsequent studies exploring associations between unemployment and a variety of illnesses and difficulties (Ferman & Gordus, 1979).

Paralleling Brenner's work was a major longitudinal study by Cobb and Kasl (1977; Kasl & Cobb, 1970; Kasl, Gore, & Cobb, 1975) examining the impact of job loss on health and mental health among 100 male blue-collar workers. This study included a comparison group of 74 workers who continued in employment (in different companies) during the study. Data collection focused on the individual worker and involved a series of home visits—which included brief physical examinations (blood and urine specimens, blood pressure, pulse rate, etc.)—and daily health diaries kept by the subjects (both employed and unemployed).

Plant-Closing Studies

In a number of cross-sectional studies during the 1970s, researchers found correlations between unemployment and a variety of health and mental health difficulties. These studies were criticized for the assumption that the direction of causality was *from* unemployment *to* deleterious health outcomes, as the reverse could equally be argued—ill health results in unemployment (Dooley & Catalano, 1988). Researchers addressed this issue during the 1980s when a series of plant closings in the United States provided opportunities to study affected workers (Buss & Redburn, 1983a, 1983b; Hamilton, Broman, Hoffman, & Renner, 1990; Perrucci, Perrucci, Targ, & Targ, 1988). It was argued that the direction of causality could be established *from* unemployment *to* subsequent deleterious health effects, as workers' ill health could not logically be viewed as the cause of the closing of a major manufacturing plant (see Dooley & Catalano, 1988).

Multiple Methods and Interests

Many of the early unemployment studies documented a number of deleterious consequences for both workers and other family members. These findings led Figley and McCubbin (1983), in their overview volume *Stress and the Family: Coping With Catastrophe,* to classify unemployment as a potentially catastrophic family stressor. More recent research, using a variety of methods and examining a number of different aspects of the unemployment experience, indicates that the answer to such questions as, "Is unemployment of a worker inevitably a family catastrophe?" may well be, "It depends."

In countries or communities where resources are made available for both support of families and retraining of workers, the transition from employment into unemployment and then into reemployment—although quite stressful at times—may not be a catastrophe at all. In fact, in some cases it may even be a welcome opportunity for change to a more satisfying job. Recent development and analysis of longitudinal nationally representative U.S. data sets—such as the Displaced Worker Survey (DWS), the Current Population Survey (CPS), the Survey of Income and Program Participation (SIPP), and the Panel Study of Income Dynamics (PSID)—provide researchers with opportunities to follow employment and unemployment patterns over time as well as to identify groups of workers who are at increased risk for long-term deleterious outcomes. In addition, recent studies have been focused on a variety of levels of outcomes, including (a) consequences of unemployment and plant closings for workers, (b) impacts on marital and family functioning, and (c) interaction of unemployment with additional stressors—and with supportive resources—in the local community and at more macro social systems levels. Theory and research findings from these diverse sources are summarized and discussed in the next two sections.

CONCEPTS, DEFINITIONS, AND THEORETICAL FRAMEWORKS

The theoretical framework most often used in studies of families and unemployment is the family stress and coping perspective. Before discussing that framework as it relates to unemployment in family systems, I offer a brief overview of definitions and some current understandings of two sets of important concepts: (a) unemployment and underemployment, and (b) deindustrialization and dislocated workers.

Unemployment and Underemployment

In discussing unemployment and families, the sociologists Mary Ann Schwartz and BarBara Scott (1994) note that the experience of unemployment can break "the complex connections between work and families" (p. 311). For the purpose of establishing unemployment rates, the U.S. government defines an *unemployed* person as one who is without a job *and* wants to work *and* has "searched for work during 4 weeks preceding the census or survey" (Korsching & Lasley, 1990). Thus, if a person has become discouraged and is no longer actively looking for a job, he or she is not counted as unemployed. Women who are homemakers are not considered employed or unemployed; their work has until recently been invisible in considerations of unemployment and the labor force.

In some studies, a person who is employed part-time but wants to work full-time is considered to be *underemployed* (rather than simply employed, as designated by the employed *or* unemployed dichotomy). Such a person may also be further subcategorized as in "involuntary part-time employment" (Schwartz & Scott, 1994, p. 314). Other subcategories of underemployment include the working poor—people who may be working full-time but because of low wages still fall below the poverty line—and persons whose current job does not fully utilize their education and skills.

Official unemployment rates—which do not recognize the category of underemployed—vary by country; by region within the United States; and by gender, age, and ethnicity. In addition, they change at least to some extent over time. As Schwartz & Scott (1994) point out, the Employment Act of 1946 (P.L. 304) and the Full Employment and Balanced Growth Act of 1978 (P.L. 95-523; 15 USC 3101) are based on the premise that there is a governmental obligation at the U.S. national system level "to use all practical means to secure the right to employment for all citizens" (p. 314). Nonetheless, U.S. unemployment rates in 1991 were 6.7% for adults, 18.6% for youth, and over 36% for black youth—both women and men (see Schwartz & Scott, 1994, p. 313).

In a discussion of unemployment theory and policy at the macro level, Brown (1983) analyzes the neoclassical economic theory that gained wide acceptance among economists and policymakers in the 1980s. According to this macrotheoretical perspective, (a) "unemployment of low-wage workers [is] not of vital concern because their productivity [is] low"; (b) "individual and social costs of unemployment . . . [are] small, since unemployed workers [have] productive alternatives—such as searching for work, doing housework, attending school, going fishing, or engaging in illegal activities"; and (c) "workers [take] advantage of the system by collecting unemployment insurance while being voluntarily unemployed" (p. 171). In contrast with a more structural approach discussed in the next section, this view is based on the assumption that an individual's unemployment is "voluntary and rational" (p. 184)—that is, the individual is free to choose whether or not he or she is unemployed. In this view, higher or lower rates of unemployment are "acceptable" (p. 184), based on the aggregate choices of free and rational individuals.

Deindustrialization and Dislocated Workers

During the late 1980s, an opposing macrotheoretical view of unemployment emerged with such concepts as *deindustrialization* and *dislocated workers.* The term deindustrialization has been used to describe the aggregate loss in the 1970s and 1980s of stable high-wage unionized manufacturing jobs—for example, in the steel and auto industries—and their replacement with low-wage, often part-time jobs with few or no benefits—for example, no health insurance or pension—often in the retail and services sectors (Bluestone & Harrison, 1982; Perrucci et al., 1988; Staudohar & Brown, 1987; Wallace & Rothschild, 1988).

Related to this view is the concept of displaced or dislocated workers —that is, "persons who have lost long-term, stable jobs due to increased international competition and/or changing technology" (Bloom, 1987, p. 157). Estimates of the numbers of such workers vary from "several hundred thousand" (Bloom, 1987, p. 157) to "11.1 million workers displaced by plant closings [between 1981 and 1985, of which] about 5.1 million—almost half—had a minimum of three years' experience in their former jobs" (Wallace & Rothschild, 1988, p. 3). There is theoretical and empirical controversy over whether these workers will subsequently find employment and whether there are substantial wage losses for those who do find a job (Berry, Gottschalk, & Wissoker, 1988; Staudohar & Brown, 1987).

In a recent discussion of social and economic class and poverty based on an underlying social systems theoretical perspective, Rank (1994) proposes a game analogy to understand employment, unemployment, and reemployment in national social systems:

> Imagine eight chairs and ten players. The players begin to circle around the chairs until the music suddenly stops. Who fails to find a chair? If the focus is on the winners and losers of the game, some combination of luck and skill will be involved. . . . However, if the focus is on the game itself, it is quite clear that, given only eight chairs, two players are bound to lose. Even if all players were suddenly to double their speed and agility, there would still be two losers. . . . I would argue that this analogy can be applied to our economic and social systems. Given that there is unemployment, given that there are periods of recession, given that there are low-paying jobs lacking benefits, given that there is occupational segregation in the labor market . . . , someone is going to lose at this game. (pp. 183-184)

Related to this approach for understanding employment and unemployment is Ferman and Gardner's (1979) discussion of the "dual labor market" (p. 201). In this view, "primary employment" encompasses full-time jobs at adequate wage levels, whereas "secondary employment" is characterized by "a reservoir of undesirable, low-paying jobs that require little or no education, skills, or experience" (p. 201). Furthermore, "laborers who hold [these jobs in the secondary labor market] constantly bounce between employment, unemployment, and nonparticipation" (p. 201).

The experience of unemployment may be very different for a previously stably employed worker who has recently been laid off in the primary labor market, versus a worker who has experienced years of secondary employment. There are also continuing empirical questions of whether—and, if so, at what cost for workers and their families—the primary labor market is losing job slots ("chairs" in Rank's, 1994, analogy) related to structural economic changes at both global and U.S. national social systems levels.

A Family Stress and Coping View of Unemployment

ABCX Model. The family systems stress and coping model has been used extensively in empirical studies of unemployment and the family (for recent reviews, see Aldous & Tuttle, 1988; Jackson & Walsh, 1987). In Figley and McCubbin's (1983) overview volume *Stress and the Family: Coping With Catastrophe,* Voydanoff (1983) uses the ABCX model as an organizing framework for understanding empirical findings regarding relationships between an unemployment event and family member outcomes. (For a general summary of the ABCX model, see Chapter 2.) Voydanoff (1983) highlights the importance of examining the event of unemployment in the context of (a) unemployment rates in the community—and therefore opportunities for subsequent reemployment—and (b) the worker's gender, age, race, and skill level —which could include the fit between the worker's skill level and reemployment opportunities in the local community social system. Also important to explore is family vulnerability to (a) financial hardship—signaled by a severe income drop (i.e., 30% or more) as well as any decrease that results in the family having income at or below the poverty threshold for family size— and (b) loss of the earner role within the family system. Outcomes of the crisis for workers and for other family members can include increased health and mental health problems as well as family instability, disruption, or violence.

Mediating factors discussed by Voydanoff (1983) include family resources and family definitions of the unemployment event. Family resources involve (a) financial resources; (b) family social system characteristics such as "adaptability, cohesion, and authority patterns" (p. 95); and (c) social supports. Aspects of the family's definition of the event include (a) suddenness—and therefore whether the family had time for preparation and anticipatory coping; (b) attribution of responsibility (particularly whether the unemployed person or other family members blame the worker for the layoff); and (c) whether the former worker experiences a sense of failure in the role of family provider. Other important coping factors are (a) whether family employment patterns can change to realign work efforts (e.g., labor force participation by additional family members); (b) effective financial management of reduced income resources; (c) the quality of family relationships, particularly with regard to flexibility of role assignments; (d) effective use of social supports, especially to reduce possible isolation and to elicit appropriate concrete resources, such as job leads, child care, and so forth; and (e) effective management of family beliefs, such as reduction of self-blame and affirmation of necessary role changes. In this view, an answer to the question of whether unemployment will be a catastrophic event for a particular family and its members is an equivocal, "It depends."

Family Transition. In addition to the ABCX model of factors for understanding the impact of an unemployment event, the family stress and coping framework incorporates a "family transition"—or roller-coaster adjustment—approach that calls attention to the likelihood that unemployment will precipitate a period of disequilibrium and change. A number of family system outcomes are possible, including recovery, maladaptation, or bonadaptation (see Chapter 2). How long this process of "realignment of family functions" takes has not been established empirically (Liem, 1985, p. 117). It is interesting to note that reemployment followed by subsequent reexperience of job loss may be *more* stressful than *stable un*employment (Ferman & Gardner, 1979, pp. 215-216). Theoretically, this could be understood in terms of multiple transitions and thus repeated or ongoing system disequilibrium.

Stress Pileup. The concept of *stress pileup* is an important but relatively recent addition to the stress and coping framework. In understanding relationships between unemployment and family system functioning, a key component has been shown to be whether the unemployment event is accompanied by additional stressors, such as economic deprivation or strain, or employment uncertainty or instability (Voydanoff, 1991, pp. 432-434; see also Ferman & Gardner, 1979). In this view, it is not the presence or absence of one event—that is, unemployment—that is key to understanding family system and family member outcomes but the event *plus* any additional prior, attendant, or subsequent stressors. Additional stressors might include poverty, marital conflict, alcohol or drug abuse, violence, or chronic unemployment that together can result in family maladaptation and deleterious consequences for individual family members.

Larger Social Systems. The family systems stress and coping model also implies the importance of attention to resources, opportunities, and constraints in larger social systems. For a family affected by an unemployment event in a larger-system environment in which job opportunities are plentiful and there is a good fit between the jobs available and the skills of the laid-off family member, the transition from employment into unemployment and subsequent reemployment may be only moderately stressful, followed by a full recovery. Even in situations where there is not a good fit between jobs in larger systems and the laid-off worker's skills, but there are financial supports as well as job retraining opportunities that are linked to actual well-paying jobs, the transition to reemployment may be somewhat more lengthy but may not require radical reorganizations in the family system. Such a supported transition may even result in greater worker satisfaction and bonadaptive consequences for family system functioning and individual family members' health and well-being.

On the other hand, where the transition involves a permanent reduction in earnings for the family provider, perhaps leading to reorganization of family roles that include two or more family members' having to be involved in employed work, the success of the new arrangements is likely to depend on the availability of stable and affordable nonparental child care, youth supervision, and other dependent care arrangements in the neighborhood or local community systems. Success may also depend on family members' ability to change perhaps long-held attitudes and beliefs about family work responsibilities (Rubin, 1976). As discussed in Chapter 4, changes in global and national economic systems have resulted in increasing numbers of U.S. families finding it necessary to have two adults in full-time employed work to meet expected family expenditures. In situations where unemployment means increased vulnerability to poverty-level wages, including patterns of unstable reemployment or chronic unemployment, the potential for family maladaptation and even catastrophe is likely to be greatly increased. Based on these theoretical understandings, in the following section, I summarize current empirical knowledge regarding relationships between unemployment and family conditions.

CURRENT RESEARCH FINDINGS

There has been a virtual explosion of unemployment research in the past decade. In this section, I present and briefly discuss (a) findings from countries other than the United States; (b) U.S. studies focusing on larger systems, such as community changes and regional trends; (c) impacts of unemployment on individual workers, including identification of demographic characteristics such as age, gender, race, and ethnicity that are associated with greater risk for deleterious consequences; (d) consequences of job loss on subsequent earnings and labor force participation; (e) impacts and interaction of unemployment with marital and family functioning, including consequences for children; and (f) associations between job loss and family dissolution as well as between unemployment and initial family formation.

Findings From Other Countries

Because findings from countries other than the United States are not directly generalizable to U.S. individuals, families, or larger social systems (e.g., neighborhoods, local communities, states, or the nation), I discuss these studies separately. These findings may have relevance for understanding various aspects of a general relationship between unemployment and families, however—understandings that will then need to be empirically examined specifically with regard to a U.S. context.

Recent comprehensive literature reviews in the United Kingdom have established a number of deleterious health (Smith, 1987) and mental health (Warr, 1987) outcomes of unemployment for many individual workers. In these reviews and additional emerging research, it was also noted, however, that the unemployment event or experience may not be the "cause" (Kagan, 1987) or key factor in understanding ill health, depression, or specific symptoms, because both unemployment *and employment* can be "good" or "bad" (Warr, 1987, p. vii). In fact, certain kinds of employment can have significant deleterious health consequences.

A New Zealand study (Hesketh, Shouksmith, & Kang, 1987) empirically identified groups of "happy" and "unhappy" employed and unemployed workers. Unhappy employed workers noted, among other things, that the "job does not use [my] skills and abilities" and that "co-workers on the job [are] unpleasant" (p. 177). In contrast, the typical happy unemployed worker was "engaged in purposeful activity (i.e., unpaid work)," was "able to help [his] wife care for [the] children" and had "good social contacts through church, etc." (p. 177).

In a Danish study, Iversen and Sabroe (1988) found that change —from employment to unemployment, *or* from unemployment to employment—was stressful for shipyard workers and that "fear of unemployment [among *employed* workers] was strongly associated with reduced psychological well-being" (p. 141). (For a U.S. study of the impact of job insecurity on marital and family relationships, see Larson, Wilson, & Beley, 1994.) In a study of older unemployed blue-collar workers in the Federal Republic of Germany, Frese (1987) found that workers "whose hopes [of finding a job] are [over time] destroyed by reality become depressed" (p. 214); this author recommends offering such workers early retirement and increased financial support.

Grayson (1986) explored changes in political attitudes among Canadian workers affected by plant closings and found, "Former employees and their spouses had less faith in their ability to affect the political process than the general population" (p. 332). They "were no more likely than the general population to opt for radical means of change" (p. 332), however—such as occupying their workplaces or seizing control of production from management (p. 333). This author notes the importance of examining empirically "how cultural, community, and institutional contexts mediate the experience of job loss (including, for example, the study of social safety nets)" (p. 333).

A variety of factors have been identified as keys to understanding associations found between unemployment and ill health and mental illness. These include attitudes toward work and work identity—e.g., job loss as "a major identity loss" among Swedish shipyard workers (Joelson & Wahlquist, 1987); economic hardship (Grayson, 1985); and "poverty, poor housing, environment, poor nutrition, etc." (Smith, 1987, p. vi). As noted previously, these findings may or may not directly apply to U.S. workers' experiences with unemployment. They do indicate possible useful areas for future exploration, however, including the need to examine consequences for individual workers in the context of the functioning of various types of larger social systems and structures.

Larger-System Impacts and Interactions

Some studies in the United States in the past decade have been focused on national economic trends and their impact on and interaction with changes in the functioning of regional and community social systems. Using national U.S. government data, Hansen (1988) discusses the displacement of workers from manufacturing jobs and notes that although new jobs are being created in the service sector, out of 470,000 new jobs generated in July 1987, "324,000 of them were part-time jobs filled by 'persons who want full-time jobs'" (p. 157). Older, less-educated workers with higher seniority in their former jobs are most at risk for large earnings losses in new employment— particularly if they are reemployed in a different occupation or industry (see also Howland

& Peterson, 1988). In addition, earnings losses "were greatest in areas of high unemployment and small labor markets" (Hansen, 1988, p. 156).

In a study of regional issues related to plant closings and worker displacement, Howland (1988) found, "Approximately 2.6 million manufacturing workers, with previously stable work histories, were involuntarily and permanently laid off between 1981 and 1986" (p. 2). In addition, she notes, "Communities can also face difficult adjustments after a plant closing or mass layoff. When a large employer closes or downsizes, local governments can be hit with a declining tax base, a rising tax burden, and reductions in the quality of services" (p. 2). A belief that problems of displacement for workers and their families can and should be addressed solely at the local level is often unrealistic. Howland (1988) concludes, "Worker displacement is a national issue" (p. 11) and calls for specific federal policies to address both individual and community difficulties.

In other studies, researchers have examined local community impacts from and responses to unemployment from a major plant closing. Officials in some communities have attempted to keep plants from closing by offering incentives such as reductions in utility costs and taxes (Perrucci et al., 1985). Following closings, not only were the unemployed workers affected, but other businesses suffered "ripple effect" losses because former workers and their families had less money to spend (e.g., in grocery stores, clothing stores, restaurants; for doctors and other medical care professionals; and in drugstores and other general merchandise businesses). Losses were also incurred because supplies and services the company had purchased locally were no longer required (Perrucci et al., 1988).

Other studies have documented "the breakdown in community life once rooted in the mills of New England" (Wagner, 1991, p. 15) and the exodus of young people from communities with high unemployment. Loss of jobs further weakens the likelihood of outside investment and community viability (Biegel, Cunningham, Yamatani, & Martz, 1989). Compounding these problems is the hesitancy of some families to use traditional community organizations and agencies for the help they may need, particularly health and mental health services (Biegel et al., 1989; see also Buss & Redburn, 1983a). Biegel and his colleagues (1989) argue for both local action initiatives and social work advocacy efforts at state and national levels "to address issues of economic growth, job security, and worker benefits" (p. 406). A multilevel social systems approach is emerging as key both to understanding current unemployment trends and effects and to addressing individual and family difficulties.

Consequences for Individual Workers

A number of reviews of U.S. unemployment research—including plant-closing studies—have documented deleterious health and mental health consequences of unemployment for laid-off workers (Briar, 1988; Gordus, Jarley, & Ferman, 1981; Jones, 1988; Liem & Rayman, 1982; Perrucci et al., 1988; Vosler, 1994). Individual difficulties associated with job loss include increased substance or alcohol use; headaches; gastrointestinal, heart, and respiratory problems; and high blood pressure (Perrucci et al., 1988) as well as significantly higher levels of depression, anxiety, and somatization (Kessler, Turner, & House, 1987).

On the other hand, recent studies have also shown "adverse effects [i.e., significant elevations of depression, anxiety, somatization and self-reported physical illness among the currently unemployed] were largely reversed by re-employment" (Kessler, Turner, & House, 1988, p. 69; see also Kessler, Turner, & House, 1989). These researchers empirically identified "social support (as measured by social integration and the availability of a confidant), [positive] self-concept, and various coping processes [such as cutting back on expenses, and use of public assistance]" as having important modifying effects on health and mental health outcomes for unemployed workers (Turner, Kessler, & House, 1991, p. 521). These scholars also empirically demonstrate that, for southeastern Michigan, "The effect of job loss on several health outcomes involves two mechanisms: (1) unemployment results in increased financial strain which, in turn, results in negative health effects, and (2) unemployment leaves the individual more vulnerable to the impact of unrelated life events [such as marital or other interpersonal relationship problems]" (Kessler et al., 1987, p. 949).

In a study of workers experiencing unemployment due to a plant closing, Beckett (1988) concluded that the provision of adequate economic supports—severance payments, pension benefits, social security, unemployment benefits—buffered the impact of the layoff on mental and physical health. Similarly, Figueira-McDonough (1978) found that availability of "concrete help for everyday needs" was "the most important buffer to psychological strain for the unemployed subjects in the study" (p. 383).

Liem and Liem's (1988) findings demonstrate, "Unemployment cannot be treated only as a personal event" (p. 96), especially among male workers who are also husbands and fathers. Using longitudinal data, these researchers found, "Involuntary unemployment created significant increases in emotional strain" both in the short term and following a year of continuing unemployment. They identified a "critical period [after 6 months of unemployment], at which time various accommodations to the loss of work appear to have prevented further elevations in psychological distress among some couples" (p. 96). Such accommodations might include role shifts between the spouses or new patterns of financial coping.

Hamilton, Hoffman, Broman, and Rauma (1993), in a 2-year longitudinal plant-closings study, found that not only did unemployment predict depression one year later, but depression one year after a plant closing, in turn predicted unemployment for 2 years after the plant closing. Thus, "The results are consistent with the argument that just as unemployment leads to depression, depression itself leads to unemployment" (p. 240).

Using a different set of research questions, a number of researchers have identified groups of workers particularly vulnerable to unemployment or to particularly negative outcomes from an unemployment event. In a study of worker displacement (defined as "job loss among workers with significant labor-force attachment"), Hamermesh (1989) concluded, "Minorities suffer an above-average rate of displacement (p. 1989). In addition, "Less-educated workers spend more time unemployed and suffer disproportionate wage losses" (p. 58). Furthermore, Hamilton et al. (1990) found, "For the low-income, the less educated, and especially the less educated black worker, the mental health impact [i.e., more depression, higher anxiety] of layoff was profound" (p. 136). In a study of unemployed black adults, Brown and Gary (1985) found, "Depressive symptoms are less among unemployed persons with higher levels of income, education, religiosity, age and satisfactory social support" (p. 736).

In a study of unemployment and reemployment, Jones (1991b) found, "Only about 35% of those 40 [years of age] or older found work in the 15 week period [of the study] while 60% of those under 40 returned to work. It may be assumed since education, skills, and occupations were similar for both groups, that ageism might be a factor in whether one found new work" (p. 12). On the other hand, in a study of unemployed autoworkers affected by plant closings, Hoffman, Hamilton, Broman, and Rauma (1991) found that younger workers were more depressed.

Only a few studies have examined unemployment among women workers. Using focus group discussion with 61 low-income women who had lost their jobs in the previous 6 months, Donovan, Jaffe, and Pirie (1987) identified "five areas that nearly all the women regarded as critical to their ability to cope with the loss of employment . . . (1) loss of income, (2) loss of fulfillment and self-esteem, (3) strain on the family, (4) loss of social support from the workplace, and (5) time management/ loss of structure and purpose" (p. 302). Jones (1989) found, "A woman's reaction to unemployment appears to hinge on the degree of financial distress that joblessness creates for her and on the meaning of work she assigns for herself" (p. 64).

In a study of laid-off autoworkers, Hoffman, Hamilton, et al. (1991) found that the unemployed women were more depressed than the men. In an examination of gender differences in the effects of unemployment on psychological distress, Ensminger and Celentano (1990) found evidence to "suggest that when gender differences in psychological distress are found they may be due to differences in role configurations [e.g., parenting responsibilities, responsibility for finances, perceived lack of social support] of men and women rather than intrinsic gender differences" (p. 469).

Reemployment and Earnings

As noted above, two critical factors in understanding the impact of unemployment on health and mental health of workers are subsequent employment status (reemployment versus long-term unemployment) and financial strain. In a study of job search outcomes, using data from the Survey of Income and Program Participation, it was found that overall 67.4% of job searches resulted in the job seeker finding a job (U.S. Bureau of the Census, 1989, p. 11). The percentages for finding a job (versus "withdrew") were higher for white men (aged 20 to 24: 86.7%; aged 25 to 54: 85.0%), lower for white women (62.8%), and dramatically lower for all blacks (52.7%), black men aged 20 to 24 (58.2%), black women (44.6%), all Hispanics (57.8%), and Hispanic women (43.2%) (p. 11).

With regard to reemployment earnings and wage loss, Madden (1988) found, "Blue collar workers, industry changers, white women, and black men who are displaced incur the greater losses" (p. 93). Berry et al. (1988) found "a sharp increase in the proportion of persons with earnings below $10,000" during a period of displacement (p. 702). On the other hand, they suggest, "If the distributional concern is to avoid large increases in the proportion of persons with low earnings then there is a short-term problem but one that seems to dissipate over time" (p. 706). They also empirically describe an income "disadvantaged individual" as "a 25-year old, non-union black household head with 12 years of schooling" (p. 706). In addition to at least some short-term earnings losses, "Most displaced workers lose employer-financed health insurance along with their jobs" (Podgursky & Swaim, 1987, p. 30). These authors further note that their data "suggest that such workers ran a high risk of remaining uninsured for extended periods, even after new employment was secured" (p. 30).

Family Impacts and Interactions

In a number of recent studies, researchers have paid particular attention to the impact of unemployment on other members of the laid-off worker's family—such as spouse or children—as well as on family interaction patterns.

In their analysis of longitudinal data from adults who grew up during the Depression, Elder and Rockwell (1985) comment on "the importance of the parental marriage for the well-being of children in crisis situations" (p. 53). They note in particular that economic deprivation in childhood due to parental unemployment was predictive of psychosocial difficulties in adulthood—for example, anxiety, lack of energy, heavy drinking—and that this association was exacerbated when the child had grown up in the midst of a divisive parental marriage. As Elder and others point out, "Economic change disrupts customary ways of living and behaving" (Liker & Elder, 1983, p. 350). This results in disequilibrium and change for all members of the family system. On the other hand, family support, including a cohesive marriage, can buffer negative effects of unemployment on individual workers and in some situations can even provide a supportive environment in which positive change becomes possible (Gordus et al., 1981).

Rook, Dooley, and Catalano (1991) found, "Husbands' job stressors [including job loss] were associated with elevated psychological distress among their wives" (p. 171). These authors recommend future empirical examination of "interdependent reactions of a couple to stressful life events" (p. 175) rather than focusing exclusively on one individual (i.e., the unemployed person) in a family.

Robertson, Elder, Skinner, and Conger (1991) found evidence for the importance of examining whether husbands had a stable—versus an unstable—work history. Their results indicated that in families headed by a man with an unstable work history, "The wife's support from external sources [relatives and friends] ameliorates her distress but it can also affirm the husband's sense of failure as a breadwinner" (p. 403) and "may intensify marital discord and increase the risk of paternal punitiveness" (p. 413).

In a number of studies, financial strain and economic hardship have been found to be keys in understanding both individual and family outcomes of unemployment (Broman, Hamilton, & Hoffman, 1990; Conger et al., 1990; Elder & Caspi, 1988; Hoffman, Carpentier-Alting, Thomas, Hamilton, & Broman, 1991; Liem & Liem, 1988; Liker & Elder, 1983; Pearlin & Turner, 1987). As will be discussed further in Chapter 8, stress pileup from the combination of chronic unemployment and poverty can destabilize family relationships and adversely affect all members of a family system.

Recent studies have found strong evidence of an association linking unemployment, financial strain, and marital and family conflict. Dail (1988) found that for unemployed families, the problems most frequently reported were (a) "increased strain to meet costs of food, clothing, and energy"; (b) "increased strain to meet medical/dental expenses"; (c) "increase in number of issues remaining unresolved"; (d) "increased conflict between husband and wife"; and (e) "increased conflict between parents and children" (p. 32).

Broman et al. (1990) conclude, "Results indicate that financial hardship produced by the unemployment experience has powerful negative effects on . . . families" (p. 643). In particular, these two experiences (unemployment and financial hardship) in combination predict higher levels of marital tension and conflict as well as increased likelihood of parent-child conflict—including fathers reporting "hitting and slapping" their children (p. 653).

Liem and Liem (1988) found that a strong marital relationship can buffer adverse psychological effects of unemployment on workers and their wives. On the other hand, in families in which unemployment resulted in changes in the provider role—for example, where the woman went back to work or increased her work hours—changes in role relationships can result in family conflict (Aldous & Tuttle, 1988). In addition, "Marital conflict was especially high if wives got jobs for the first time" (p. 34).

In a review of studies of the effects of plant closings and unemployment on families, Targ and Perrucci (1990) note, "Parents' responses to unemployment may include anger, hostility, and even abuse of their children. . . . The greater the economic hardship that displaced parents perceived they were experiencing, the greater their hostility. Moreover, the greater these parents' hostility, the more their oldest child had problems at home" (pp. 137-138). Jones (1991a) found that a number of factors influenced the impact of unemployment on the father-child relationship. These included (a) "the father's reaction to job loss" (e.g., irritability, frustration, perceived loss of power), (b) the "mother's reaction to job loss" (e.g., feelings about entry into the workforce, reaction to role changes, whether she blames her husband for the job loss), and (c) "characteristics of the child" (e.g., age and gender) (p. 103; see also Jones, 1990).

Flanagan (1990) found that adolescents—especially boys—"in deprived households [defined as reported parental layoff or demotion, with no subsequent reemployment] . . . reported the highest conflict with parents" in comparison with adolescents in families with stable employment or with work loss but subsequent reemployment (p. 163). Their findings "suggest that conflict with parents intensifies for adolescent boys when parents are 'unavailable' due to a lack of family strengths or to parents' preoccupation with changing employment conditions" (p. 174). On the other hand, "Mothers in deprived households reported that they granted their daughters more autonomy than they granted their sons," resulting in less conflict (p. 174).

In summary, studies indicate that no one factor is decisive in understanding relationships between unemployment, families, and individual family members. Instead, an examination of multiple factors over time —including an exploration of stress pileup—is key to developing a comprehensive picture (Voydanoff, 1991). In work with families experiencing the potentially catastrophic stress of unemployment, a multilevel model, such as that depicted in Figure 6.1, is essential in identifying specific stressors and resources as well as potential change points. Based on the family stress and coping framework, including the family system disequilibrium and transition understanding of adaptation to a stressful event such as unemployment, the model in Figure 6.1 specifically directs practitioners' and family members' attention to (a) prior-to-unemployment family characteristics; (b) formal (outside of the family) and family (internal) resources; (c) family definitions and coping strategies; (d) worker experience with job search and reemployment; (e) family economic change and hardship; (f) possible role changes and family members' perceptions of these changes (such as the necessity to shift

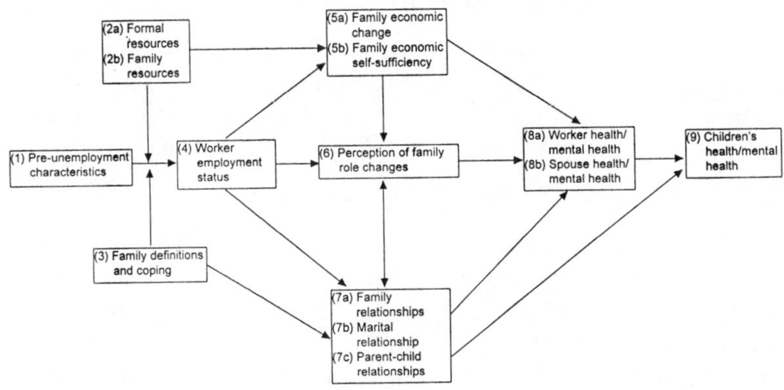

Figure 6.1. Key Factors for Understanding Laid-Off Workers and Their Families

SOURCE: Vosler (1994, p. 10). Copyright 1994 by Families International, Inc. Reprinted by permission.

from one provider to two providers and the accompanying risk of role overload); (g) family, marital, and parent-child relationships; and (h) worker and spouse health and mental health—which over time are likely to be highly predictive of (i) children's health and mental health outcomes.

As noted in a previous discussion of this model (Vosler, 1994) and discussed in detail in Chapter 7, direct service practitioners may be able to assist some families with internal role changes to help the family adapt to the need for two providers for family economic self-sufficiency. Unless there are jobs available for reemployment, however, as well as resources in the community to provide any needed retraining and to support the complexity of balancing employed work and family work roles (see Chapter 4), then practitioners—as well as the families affected by unemployment and changes in the economy—are likely to confront frustration of their goal of stable, healthy family life. Inability to reach the goal of family health is particularly likely if continuing unemployment, or low-wage employment, results in the family's sliding into poverty—and the often-associated reality of destabilizing stress pileup.

Family Formation and Dissolution

In addition to examining the impact of unemployment on family members' health and on the healthy functioning of families as systems, researchers have begun to explore possible associations between unemployment and family formation and dissolution. Particularly in these areas, the impact of unemployment and poverty *in combination* seems critical.

As Voydanoff (1991) notes, "A minimum level of income and employment stability is necessary for family stability and cohesion. Without it, many are unable to form families through marriage and others find themselves subject to separation and divorce" (p. 435). Without stable employment that produces income adequate to cover the needs of the family, individuals may delay marriage (see Chadiha, 1992) or may not marry at all. Among married workers, unemployment has been found to be associated with increased risk for separation and divorce (Voydanoff, 1991).

Wilkie (1991) found, "Men's, especially young men's, ability to support families has been declining since the mid-1960s . . . [which] is associated with a decrease in the marriage rate of young men, a rise in the proportion of young mothers who do not marry, and a decline in marital fertility" (p. 119). She also suggests, "Men's declining earning power may indirectly contribute to the rise in the proportion of families with no male present by increasing the risk of divorce and separation" (p. 119).

In summary, although unemployment does not necessarily or inevitably lead to deleterious consequences for families or for individual family members, the experience of unemployment must be considered a risk factor for negative outcomes—particularly when associated with economic hardship and financial strain. In addition, recent research indicates that unemployment or the inability to earn enough income to support a family may negatively affect families by delaying or inhibiting initial family formation as well as by increasing the risk of parental separation or divorce.

SUMMARY

Increasingly, research and theory have demonstrated that the experience of layoff and unemployment is not only an individual event but involves other family members and changes family system relationships and functioning. A multilevel view of current unemployment enables practitioners to examine a family's experience of an unemployment event in the context of local employment and unemployment realities and larger-system policies and services—or lack of these—for supporting workers and their families in the transition to stable reemployment (or unstable reemployment-unemployment cycles, retirement, etc.).

A great deal more knowledge is critically needed for understanding the structural economic changes currently under way at national, state, and local levels, and how economic changes at the global level impact these changes. If large numbers of job slots ("chairs," in Rank's, 1994, metaphor) are being permanently lost in the primary labor market, this change has the potential for dramatic negative effects on the formation and stable functioning of large numbers of families.

In addition, more research is needed for understanding how short- or long-term participation in the secondary labor market affects both family formation and family stability. Findings from current studies suggest that where employment is unstable—with the necessity for constant family reorganization around a changing provider role or roles—and particularly where wages are low and also unstable, family formation may be delayed or may never occur. Families that do form may experience a pileup of stress that can lead to separation and divorce.

Much more knowledge also is needed regarding economic development at local, state, and national system levels and family social supports. Understandings are critical regarding socioeconomic development at multiple levels, including jobs development, wages, benefits, and income supports, to ensure that family members can adequately fulfill the provider role or roles. In addition, knowledge is needed regarding effective supports to enable family members to make the transition to stable employment—at wages that provide adequately for basic family needs—along with neighborhood and community services (such as child care, sick care, youth supervision, etc.) to enable parents to fulfill both employed work and family work responsibilities. At the neighborhood and local levels, critical supports are likely to include job training or retraining, transitional income supports, and a variety of family and other services to ensure that parents are able to balance participation in the labor force with the critical role of raising the next generation.

Social work practitioners and researchers are in a strong position to make major contributions in the development of critically needed policies and services at neighborhood, local, state, and national levels. They also must participate in the development of empirically based knowledge regarding what is effective, for whom, and with what costs and benefits. In particular, understandings of "the game(s)" of employment and unemployment, wages, and supports for families—and particularly for families traditionally disadvantaged in the labor market, such as men of color and women—must begin to trace the long-term social costs of ignoring issues of discrimination and disruptive structural economic change. It is imperative that as a nation, the United States move beyond an individualistic understanding of "family problems" to confront the difficult issues of employed work as family provision in balance with family work. Voters—including social workers and other human service professionals—must address the social choices and decisions that are necessary for the development of stable family systems and healthy parents and children.

Chapter 7

FAMILIES AND UNEMPLOYMENT
Applications and Tools for Practice

CASE SUMMARY

To update the situation of the Smith family (see Chapter 5), Figure 7.1 presents an overview of the family in 1995 and Figure 7.2 delineates Peter and Jane Smith's household time and tasks plan (see also Figure 3.6 and Figures 5.1 and 5.2). In 1993, the Smith family began work with a social worker provided by an Employee Assistance Program (EAP) through Peter's union. Later in 1993, the auto assembly plant where Peter had worked for the previous 5 years closed.

Until several weeks after the actual plant closing, Peter believed that somehow the union would be able to "save" his and his friends' jobs. But after several months of seeing Marvin, the EAP worker, Peter began to talk about the possibility of taking an auto mechanics course offered through the retraining program set up jointly by the plant and the union. He and Jane were able to discuss with Marvin the fact that a job in this field might provide much lower wages than his auto assembly job, and that Jane might have to work full-time to help make ends meet for the family.

Marvin was involved in a local community group helping to locate jobs for laid-off workers. Through these contacts, he was able, after nearly a year, to help Jane get a full-time secretarial job with the city. Because of training benefits and income from unemployment insurance—including a substantial supplemental unemployment benefit through the union—Peter was able to provide for his family as well as take a one-year course in auto repair. Marvin also helped the family negotiate with the bank to adjust their mortgage payments to their ability to pay.

INCOME:			
Net pay (after deductions):			
his:	$15,000		
hers:	$10,000		
Total:			$25,000
EXPENDITURES:			
Fixed:			
Mortgage	$ 8,400		
Day care	$ 4,500		
Insurance	$ 1,000		
Subtotal, fixed:		$13,900	
Variable:			
Food and other grocery items	$ 5,200		
Utilities	$ 1,200		
Telephone	$ 300		
Repairs	$ 500		
Automobile	$ 1,200		
Clothing and personals	$ 1,200		
Medical	$ 1,000		
Vacation	$ 500		
Subtotal, variable:		$11,100	
Total Expenses:			$25,000
TOTAL INCOME - TOTAL EXPENSES:			$ 0

Figure 7.1. 1995 Smith Family Budget (Yearly)

In addition, Marvin supported Jane in her insistence that Peter get help for his alcohol problem. At one point, Jane threatened to leave her husband if he did not get professional help for his problem drinking and his associated threats of violence toward her and the children.

While Jane was looking for a full-time job, she also searched for high-quality child care for Kevin and Susan. She finally was able to get on a waiting list at a day care center run by a nearby church, and at about the same time that she began full-time employment, two day care slots opened up for the children. Jane's mother agreed to provide backup sick care, at least until she located a job for herself. Jane recently attended a parents' group associated with the day care center, where she heard other parents discuss concerns similar to hers about backup care for sick children.

	Peter	Jane
I. Provider Roles:		
Paid job	50 hours/week (including travel)	45 hours/week (including travel)
II. Household Maintenance:		
Food/meals/nutrition	2 hours/week shopping	28 hours/week
Cleaning, etc.	1 hour/week	4 hours/week
Clothing/Other Shopping	2 hours/month (.5 hours/week)	2 hours/month (.5 hours/week)
Laundry	3 hours/week	
Repairs	2 hours/month (.5 hours/week)	
Yard	1 hour/week	
Auto maintenance	2 hours/month (.5 hours/week)	
III. Family Leadership and Decision-Making	2 hours/week	2 hours/week
IV. Dependents' Care (Including travel to and from child care)	15 hours/week	15 hours/week
V. Children and Youth Supervision and Socialization	10 hours/week	10 hours/week
Total:	85.5 hours/week	104.5 hours/week

Figure 7.2. 1995 Smith Household Time and Tasks

Following a year of training, Peter found a full-time job in his field, although it is a fairly long commute from home. Jane hopes to take a nursing course once both children are in school.

With both parents working full-time, there have been long and often intense discussions between Peter and Jane, sometimes with Marvin, about budgeting as well as how to allocate tasks within the Smith household. Jane feels more supported and less stressed now that Peter is making a good-faith effort to spend more time doing family work—including shopping, laundry, and care and supervision of the children. Marvin has supported and encouraged Peter and Jane in the major changes that they have worked out in family beliefs and patterns. He has also helped them share their accomplishments with extended-family members, including Peter's father and oldest brother and Jane's parents.

In this chapter, I focus on systemic practice with and on behalf of families experiencing the potentially catastrophic stressor event of unemployment. The chapter is organized as follows: (a) discussion of policy and program interventions and their evaluation at multiple social systems levels; (b) presentation of tools for family assessment as well as discussion of critical components of social work practice with unemployed workers and their families; and (c) delineation of strategies for social change, including advocacy, knowledge building, and development of interdisciplinary models.

MULTILEVEL INTERVENTIONS AND EVALUATION

As discussed in Chapter 6, an unemployment event is potentially, but not necessarily, a catastrophic stressor for a laid-off worker—such as Peter—and his or her family. How families such as the Smiths cope with the stress event within the family is one aspect of the overall picture. In the long term, an even more critical aspect of individual and family adaptation to changes occasioned by unemployment is the set of macrosystems components delineated in Figure 6.1: (a) "employment status" (#4), (b) family economic change and self-sufficiency (#5a & b), and (c) formal and informal resources (#2a & b). As discussed briefly in Chapter 6 and delineated in detail in Chapter 8, in families in which unemployment occasions a drop in family income below the poverty line—particularly if unemployment continues irregularly or poverty becomes chronic—the potential for catastrophic stress pileup increases dramatically in spite of family-level interventions. Consequently, identification or development of critical intervention and prevention components in larger social systems to ensure that family providers such as Peter and Jane have access to stable reemployment at adequate wages as well as appropriate transitional supports are critical. Thus, discussion of these components precedes presentation of family-level assessment tools and interventions. I delineate three multilevel intervention components: (a) accurately perceiving current economic realities, (b) developing and evaluating policies and programs, and (c) understanding various practitioner roles in context.

Perceiving Multilevel Economic Realities

To work with families such as the Smiths and devise effective programs for workers and families affected by unemployment, practitioners like Marvin must first grasp the multilevel economic realities discussed in detail in Chapter 6. In agency settings and professional organizations and associations, social workers in both clinical and policy practice must understand global socioeconomic changes and their impacts on national, state, and local economic structures and social systems.

Because of changing economic trends over the past several decades, including deindustrialization, increases in part-time jobs, and stagnant or falling wage levels for many workers in the national (U.S.) social system, an assumption by either an unemployed worker like Peter (and her or his family) or by a direct service practitioner such as Marvin that there will be a job available that is comparable to the job from which the worker has been laid off cannot be made without detailed understandings of current local, state, and national economies. For example, depending on the laid-off family member's education, training level, family circumstances, housing situation, and so forth, a critical decision about how widely to search for reemployment may need to be made fairly soon after layoff—that is, will the unemployed worker look only locally or would she or he and other family members be willing to relocate, either in the state or nationally (or internationally)?

Thus, social workers like Marvin, through discussions and planning with other social workers and other professionals must be able to utilize understandings of larger economic realities. Detailed understandings of those realities are needed—for example, unemployment rates and trends, major employers, small businesses, successes in economic development, job-training programs and placement rates—both in the practitioner's and clients' specific local community and in state and national-level social systems. Clear understandings of these realities can provide a base for effective work with families as well as for participation in development of effective programs and policies at both local and more macro state and national social system levels.

Policies and Programs: Development and Evaluation

Existing employment and unemployment policies and programs serve a limited number of individuals and families. These include unemployment insurance, education and (re)training programs, and policies at the national level that at least theoretically support full employment (see Dolgoff, Feldstein, & Skolnik, 1993). Several social work scholars have in the past decade focused professional discussion on national "employment policy options" such as tax credits and subsidies and public service employment (Sherraden, 1985b, p. 7; see also Sherraden, 1985a) as well as programs at both state and local levels, including economic development, neighborhood and community redevelopment, readily available job retraining and placement services, and income and social support for individuals and families (Briar, 1983, 1988; Briar & Knighton, 1988).

As Briar (1988) points out, a thorough community-level assessment in each affected neighborhood or local community is needed for understanding both available resources and gaps in policies and services. A local community group such as the one in which Marvin was involved can facilitate this process. Current research findings suggest, as indicated in Figure 6.1, that when there are opportunities for a laid-off family member to find stable reemployment (#4) at adequate wages for family economic self-sufficiency (#5), along with adequate resources (both income and social supports, #2) to make the individual and family transition from employment through unemployment to reemployment, then family disruption may be minimal. In addition, if the new job is more satisfying, individual (#8) and family (#7) well-being may be enhanced by the change. Alternatively, if the new job (#4) involves lower wages (#5) but other supports (#2—e.g., Peter's unemployment and retraining benefits) are available and family members can negotiate altered but satisfactory family roles (#6—e.g., a spouse such as Jane begins or increases employment), then family disruption (#7) may be minimized, and family members' well-being (#8 and #9) over the long term may even be enhanced.

The findings in Chapter 6 suggest that in at least some local communities in the current U.S. national social system, the number of jobs in the primary labor market—stable, full-time jobs paying a wage adequate for supporting a family—is declining. The jobs being created are more likely to involve low-wage, part-time or temporary employment in the secondary labor market. A few recent studies have been focused on long-term effects of shifts from primary to secondary labor market participation for workers, particularly for parents (e.g., "working-poor families"; see Chapter 8).

Program development and evaluation of, for example, job placement and retraining services need to go beyond a simple outcome question—"Did the client find a job?"—to include consideration of such aspects as number and stability of hours, level of wages and benefits, and whether employment is temporary or permanent—(that is, how long does the job last?). In addition, social workers such as Marvin in agencies and as members of professional organizations must participate in and evaluate effectiveness regarding comprehensive neighborhood and community projects that address goals of economic development and stable employment for all appropriate family members.

Zippay (1991), in a study of displaced industrial workers, notes the need for "a significant commitment to longer-term education—one similar to that made to veterans through the GI bill in the 1950s" (p. 567). She also suggests development of such services as relocation assistance, training stipends, and so forth that "would require financial and program supports from . . . corporations, unions, and the public sector" (p. 567).

Besides such employment, economic development, and retraining projects, social workers also have a direct stake in the development of programs that provide financial and social support to unemployed workers and their families, both to ameliorate current problems and to prevent family breakdown. Responding to the economic recession in the United States in the early 1980s, Krystal, Moran-Sackett, Thompson, and Cantoni (1983) described efforts by "family service agencies in a metropolitan area to develop special projects to serve unemployed persons and their families" (p. 67). Specific programs focused primarily on individual workers and members of their immediate families. The project included coordination and community awareness of programs providing help with job search activities as well as services addressing tangible financial needs, health problems, mental health difficulties, and marital and family stress-related problems.

Expanding on this project, Sunley and Sheek (1986) describe model programs that incorporate groups and group work services for the unemployed as well as both concrete and clinical service components, such as information and referral, financial help, family life education, direct job-related services, and community organization and education (p. 3). They also discuss advocacy and the incorporation of volunteers, including social work students, in work with the unemployed. Marvin's work with the bank to adjust Peter and Jane's mortgage payments so that they could continue in stable housing and work toward home ownership demonstrates the importance of effective advocacy.

There is also a need for ongoing program evaluation along with consequent program modifications and updates. Brabson and Himle (1987), in their study of perceptions of social welfare agencies in one Michigan county, found that those "responsible for planning services for the unemployed and poor . . . [were] largely unaware of the needs of this population" (p. 31). One of their recommendations is that "community planning agencies and community workers . . . encourage greater participation by the poor and unemployed in social planning activities so that their viewpoints are incorporated in the appropriate decision-making process; and to enhance . . . perception [among the unemployed and poor] that they have greater control of their destiny" (p. 32).

The Practitioner Role in Context

Given the complexity and interconnectedness of larger social systems —neighborhood, local community, state, nation, and globe—it is clear that social workers, whether in direct service—such as Marvin—or in policy practice, must find effective ways to expand the focus of their work through collaboration both with other social workers and across professional disciplines. In this section, I focus briefly on the following contexts for cooperative effort: (a) the practitioner in the agency, (b) the practitioner in the neighborhood and local community, (c) the practitioner in professional organizations and associations, and (d) the practitioner as citizen.

The Practitioner in the Agency. Most social work professionals are related to one or more organizations or agencies that employ them or indirectly fund or reimburse them for their practice of social work. The beliefs and understandings current in those agencies influence the work done by their employees, contractors, and so forth. If the agency setting is an open and healthy one, practitioners who focus on different problems and populations can begin to share appropriate data not only on specific cases but also on patterns and trends in client populations served by the agency, such as increasing unemployment and poverty, family breakdowns related to evictions and homelessness, school difficulties for children who move every 6 months or so because of family income and housing difficulties, and so forth. Marvin was employed by the union's EAP program and had a variety of contacts in the local community regarding jobs, rent and mortgage payments, retraining, substance abuse treatment, and child care.

If direct service practitioners are neighborhood based, practitioners in each neighborhood can map and share data regarding employment and unemployment patterns, training and education services, transportation, housing, schools, child care and youth supervision opportunities, and other formal and informal support services in the neighborhood. Alongside this effort, the agency can aggregate these data into local community data to identify trends as well as gaps and needs and subsequently modify existing programs or initiate new programs to meet those needs in neighborhoods and the local community as a whole.

The Practitioner in the Neighborhood and Local Community. Going beyond the specific focus of a particular organization or agency, a practitioner such as Marvin can participate in existing or emerging groups or organizations in the neighborhood and local community where most of her or his work is focused. Participating in a needs assessment; serving as consultant to a group developing additional services such as child care, sick care, youth supervision, and so forth; assisting with locating funding for a new program; or participating in evaluating current policies and programs are all ways that professional social workers can assist neighborhoods and local communities to develop healthy social structures and solutions for current social problems.

The Practitioner in Professional Organizations and Associations. Professional social work and social welfare organizations and associations, which are organized into local, state, national, and international groupings, can be vital avenues for dialogue, generation and sharing of new ideas and models, dissemination of evaluations of what works and what does not, advocacy for effective policies and programs, and monitoring negative and positive social trends at multiple social systems levels that affect citizens who are our clients.

The Practitioner as Citizen. As citizens in the social systems where we work and live, practitioners often have a firsthand understanding of the ways in which social structures negatively or positively affect the lives of fellow citizens. Although "radical" social work (Bailey & Brake, 1975; Jansson, 1994) may not be possible—or comfortable—for all practitioners, each can make his or her contribution to the social dialogue in local, state, and national political structures to "promote the general welfare of society" as delineated in the NASW Code of Ethics (NASW, 1993).

TOOLS FOR FAMILY ASSESSMENT

Clinical Assessment and Interventions

Only in the context of thorough knowledge of larger social systems—especially local community and neighborhood—realities can an effective assessment of individual and family difficulties be made (see Figure 6.1). As discussed in Chapter 5, particularly important tools for assessment with family members are (a) a family budget (Figure 5.3), (b) an employed work-family work ecomap (Figure 4.2), (c) patterns of household time and tasks management (Figure 5.4), (d) a family genogram, and (e) a family time line focused in particular on patterns and beliefs regarding employed work and family work. These five tools as filled out for the Smith family—see Figures 7.1 (budget), 5.2 (ecomap), 7.2 (time and tasks), 5.1 (genogram), and 3.6 (time line)— provide a detailed picture of a successful family transition, enabled by both larger-system resources (retraining, adequate long-term unemployment insurance, advocacy with the bank, substance abuse treatment, two "new"—for Peter and Jane—stable jobs, child care, and sick care) as well as intensive clinical family work to support and facilitate changes in family roles, organizational patterns, and beliefs.

Given research findings with unemployed workers and their families regarding such consequences as depression, family conflict, and even abuse and violence, practitioners must sensitively explore and be prepared to deal with such issues. Other clinical issues identified by Sunley and Sheek (1986) and by Briar (1988) are stress, anxiety, lowered self-esteem, grief, anger, blame, confusion, alcohol or drug abuse, family tension and breakdown, role adjustments, and suicidal tendencies.

Because employment instability and uncertainty are major stressors for families (Voydanoff, 1991)—and particularly because *stable un*employment has been found to be less stressful than *unstable re*employment (see Chapter 6)—employment planning is a critical component in work with a family such as the Smiths experiencing the unemployment of one or more family providers. Exploration of relocation, short-term or long-term retraining, and potential for shifts in roles within the family—such as from one family provider to two, or shifts in hours worked or family work roles—are critical (Briar, 1988).

In addition, exploration of extended-family, neighborhood, and local community resources—both their availability and accessibility—is a key component. Often financial and emotional supports from family and friends may be nearing exhaustion at the point that an unemployed worker or other family member is first seen by a professional. Consequently, immediate concrete services such as financial assistance and housing may be required. For some families, information and referral may be all that is needed. In communities where unemployment is relatively high and for workers with redundant skills—for example, unskilled blue-collar workers formerly in manufacturing jobs—intensive and fairly long-term assistance, including adequate income support and training in skills for jobs that are actually available in the local economy, may be required for family members such as Peter and Jane to accomplish their goal of stable reemployment and for the family to achieve a stable recovery.

For meeting the needs of unemployed workers and their families, several authors have noted the importance of (a) self-help activities, especially in a group setting, such as a job search support group or a more long-term job club (Briar, 1988, pp. 104-106); (b) family education about unemployment stresses and identifying all available resources and services (Sunley & Sheek, 1986); and (c) support from religious organizations (Brabson & Himle, 1987; Sunley & Sheek, 1986). Mobilization and management of a variety of services over a fairly lengthy transition period (2-5 years) may be critical for some families and family members to maintain the family as a viable social system and for family restabilization at a healthy level of functioning to occur.

Reciprocal Linkages to Community Resources

It is clear that not only the availability but also the quality and effectiveness of neighborhood and local community resources and services for unemployed workers and their families, such as the Smiths, are important in the family transition occasioned by an unemployment event. A currently unfounded public perception or belief may be that there are sufficient jobs at adequate wages to support a family for all who want to work. Thus, both voting citizens and policymakers have often focused primarily on local availability of job search information and time-limited unemployment insurance to ease the "temporary" transitions from employment to unemployment to reemployment. For the most part, the unemployed have not been asked to provide input into policy planning (Brabson & Himle, 1987); nor have service users routinely been asked to comment on the services they are offered or receive.

As the research review in Chapter 6 makes clear, however, the overall number of jobs with wages adequate to support a family appears to be declining, particularly through the process of deindustrialization. It seems that these job slots (or "chairs," in Rank's, 1994, metaphor) are primarily being replaced with lower-wage, often part-time or temporary jobs in the services sector, forcing many families—especially younger families with children—to become and remain "dual-earner" families (Chapter 4) with attendant risks for stress and role overload. When one of the necessary two family providers is laid off from a job, the entire complex family social system, which often includes a fragile balance of employed work and family work roles, is potentially thrown into disarray, affecting not only the individual worker but all other members of the immediate family system as well as extended-family members, friends, neighbors, and service providers. In a local community affected by major layoffs or plant closings, unemployment can affect individuals and families far beyond the initially laid-off workers (Vosler, 1994).

Consequently, social work practitioners such as Marvin must be able to look beyond particular clients—or even the social service system in a neighborhood or local community—to discuss both with families and with professionals at multiple levels the particular realities of employment and unemployment and resources and resource gaps in clients' neighborhoods as well as at community, state, national, and even international social system levels. Social systems and structures are developed and maintained by human actions. Social systems within the U.S. national system are guided, at least in part, by democratic beliefs and values. It is thus important for all members, including professionals and clients, to (a) have current and relevant information and knowledge, (b) have specific opportunities for feedback and dialogue, and (c) be able to participate in needed development and change to achieve healthy functioning of social systems at multiple levels.

Linkages between unemployed clients—workers and other family members—and community service resources need to become more reciprocal. Feedback from consumers regarding service and program strengths and weaknesses need to be automatically elicited as part of routine program evaluations. In addition, multiple opportunities for participation in community planning and development, including both economic and services development, should be offered to all citizens—specifically including unemployed workers and their families.

STRATEGIES FOR SOCIAL CHANGE

To be effective in current multilevel social systems realities, social work practitioners cannot afford to confine their focus and knowledge for practice to only one system level, whether that is an individual person, a family, or even a neighborhood or community. Although a particular practitioner may have special skills and professional experience for work in one or more particular levels of social systems, such as more micro skills with individuals and families or more macro skills with policies or local communities, all social work practitioners (whether direct practice or policy practice) have a stake in creating opportunities for collaboration to identify and utilize effective strategies for innovation and positive social change. Here, I briefly discuss three arenas for further development: (a) advocacy, empowerment, and "common well-being education"; (b) social work knowledge building; and (c) interdisciplinary dialogue and model development.

Advocacy, Empowerment, and "Common Well-Being Education"

As the negative impacts on family systems of such larger-system issues as unemployment, poverty, and discrimination have become clearer to a number of family practitioners (see Boyd-Franklin, 1989, 1993), calls for advocacy and empowerment strategies at multiple systems levels have increased (see also Solomon, 1976). Boyd-Franklin (1993) calls for empowerment through (a) bringing "a family . . . together in a group with other families in their community who are experiencing similar problems" (p. 373); (b) teaching family members to work in self-advocacy roles with workers in such agencies as "schools, hospitals, police, courts, juvenile justice systems, welfare, child protective services, housing, and mental health services" (p. 373); and (c) appropriate training for clinicians, including supervisors, that involves "helping therapists to look at themselves—at their own values, upbringing, and attitudes about race, class, and poverty" (p. 374) and skills to "advocate for change in our own agencies and clinics, communities, and local, state, and national government" (p. 375).

As part of this advocacy and empowerment work with larger social systems at multiple levels, social work practitioners at all levels—direct service workers (with individuals, families, and communities), administrators, researchers, and those in policy practice—must develop effective methods for "common well-being education"—that is, for educating all citizens in understanding and working for positive development of the social systems that make up the global society of which each is a member (a process that can be compared, by analogy, with the public health education movement). Dialogue and collaboration are necessary and can begin with professional organizations and associations, including religious coalitions interested in social justice issues; unions working on issues of job security and adequate wages and benefits; and neighborhood associations in many middle-class and working-class neighborhoods and communities concerned about education, housing, safety and crime prevention, economic development and jobs; and so forth.

Such work will require continuing networks for communication and dialogue, and collaboration that includes organizations and agencies in both the private and public sectors. Knowledge is needed regarding methods for appropriate sharing of information on, for example, trends in difficult, intractable, and emerging social problems and effective programs and strategies for problem solving and further development. By creating forums or roundtables for discussion and dialogue, social work practitioners are already seeing that unhelpful perceptions can sometimes be put aside. Contrary to some popular rhetoric, all public organizations and agencies are *not* rigid and ineffective bureaucratic nightmares lacking regard for the human faces of clients. Nor are all private sector organizations inhuman economic machines focusing exclusively on competition and the bottom line and oblivious to families and social issues.

Advocacy and empowerment must explicitly include not only making the system work for clients but also nurturing through positive change the multilevel social systems within which all citizens—professionals, clients, and consumers—work and live. Such a strategy requires the beginning development of components of "common well-being education" offerings for all citizens. Just as effective family system change eventually requires some level of cooperation between all family members, a social systems view of societies posits that over the long term, effective social change requires common beliefs, behaviors, and social patterns and structures that are shared—at least to some extent—by all system members. Shared understandings among increasing numbers of professionals as well as citizens—regarding, for example, multilevel social systems and structures; global socioeconomic changes; inadequacies in current policies and programs; and stressors for families and family members from employed work and family work role overload, unemployment, and poverty—could and hopefully will, over time, lead to service innovations, ongoing knowledge building, and more effective social and economic policies and programs.

Social Work Knowledge Building

As noted in Chapters 1 and 2, ongoing multilevel social systems "development" requires a continual process of professional knowledge building. Such knowledge building involves not only the gathering and sharing of valid and reliable data but also—and often equally or even more important—the ability to synthesize varieties of data into (a) usable theories for guiding program development; and (b) theory-based models for professional practice involving assessment, interventions, and evaluation.

Rothman and his colleagues (Rothman & Thomas, 1994) discuss the process of "intervention research" for designing, evaluating, and further developing programs and intervention models in the human services with the complementary goals of (a) "intervention knowledge development," and (b) knowledge utilization. Included in this discussion are "conceptual integration methods," for example, "systematic research synthesis" (Rothman, Damron-Rodriguez, & Shenassa, 1994, p. 137), designed to enhance the growth of knowledge for practice. Also discussed are (a) "fostering participation" (Rothman, Teresa, & Erlich, 1994, p. 377), (b) "interorganizational exchange" (Hasenfeld & Furman, 1994), and (c) "dissemination" of treatment innovations (Corrigan, MacKain, & Liberman, 1994, p. 317).

Especially with regard to such large-scale economic systems issues as unemployment and deindustrialization, it is clear that continuing documentation of negative—as well as positive—consequences of changes in structures and patterns for both individuals and family systems is a critical component in understanding and proposing changes in current policies and programs. In addition to intervention research, there is a need for development of neighborhood and community social systems tools and methods that bring together a comprehensive picture, including economic, political, and cultural structures and subsystems, of the strengths and needs of a particular social system, whether neighborhood, community, state, or nation.

Included in this documentation of trends and consequences must be the development of valid and reliable methods for calculating the social and economic costs of not responding to negative economic changes and social difficulties. For example, there are individual and family costs of family providers experiencing—within larger social systems—employment instability or employment uncertainty or both (Voydanoff, 1991). Such costs include lower marital satisfaction, increased family stress, and possible health and mental health difficulties. Professional knowledge development efforts must begin to track, at individual and family levels and at larger-system levels, the social, emotional, and health consequences and subsequent costs (e.g., in substance abuse and addiction, child abuse and domestic violence, unsafe neighborhoods and schools, and need for additional health and mental health services as well as costly child welfare services) of *not* addressing the issue of stable employment at wages and benefits adequate to support stable family systems.

Interdisciplinary Dialogue and Model Development

Development of theory, models, and proposals for policies and programs to achieve positive social systems change will need to be carried out with the cooperation of both service users and professionals in collaborative efforts that cross traditional boundaries separating disciplines and professions, and professionals and clients. For example, "solving" problems of families with unemployed or underemployed family providers involves not only working with family members regarding roles, communication, managing resources, and so forth, but necessitates the development in the neighborhood and local community of comprehensive and effective economic, transportation, and services systems that ensure every family's access to adequate housing; education; child, dependents, and sick care; health care; recreation and youth supervision services; and so forth. Such efforts need to involve not only a variety of theoretical disciplines—economics, political science, sociology, anthropology, psychology—but also a diversity of professionals, including social workers, educators, health care providers, businesspersons, legislators, planners, architects, engineers, and others.

At the macrosystems levels of state and nation, development and implementation of viable policy models for addressing the need for full employment (Briar, 1988; Sherraden, 1985a, 1985b; Voydanoff, 1987) require common understandings and cooperation between policy practice professionals and citizens as voters. Scholars from a variety of disciplines have articulated the need for comprehensive family policy initiatives (Chilman, 1988a; Googins, 1991; Hartman, 1993; Kamerman, 1986; Moen, 1992; Voydanoff, 1987; Zimmerman, 1992). Long-term cooperation and the development of mutual understandings of issues—as well as of common goals and strategies—are necessary for the creation of substantial social changes. Understanding of options and alternatives, and of potential costs and consequences, are needed, based on current theory, research, and practice models. Proposals for needed change can be drawn from experiences both within the U.S. national social system and from other countries in the larger social system of Planet Earth—for example, from Sweden and other European countries; countries redeveloped following the devastation of World War II, such as Japan; rural communities; developing countries; urban neighborhoods; and multiethnic city-states (such as Singapore and Hong Kong).

SUMMARY

To be effective in work with families experiencing the potentially catastrophic stress of unemployment, workers often must focus beyond assessment and interventions in the family system; they must be able to see current multilevel economic realities and trends and must assess and work to develop needed programs and policies, particularly in their agency's neighborhood and local community, through participation in professional organizations and associations as well as through activities as citizens. In a changing economic environment, continuing feedback from clients as well as from local citizens is likely to be needed to develop effective programs and services. In addition, strategies for change at larger systems levels are required, including (a) advocacy, empowerment, and "common well-being education"; (b) continual social work knowledge building; and (c) interdisciplinary dialogue and model development.

Chapter 8

FAMILIES AND POVERTY
Theory and Research

As discussed in Chapter 6, an unemployment event in and of itself does not inevitably result in deleterious consequences for families—and may even lead to enhanced opportunities. But when unemployment is combined with economic hardship, and particularly when one or both factors last longer than a brief period, then the risk of negative outcomes for family members and for the family as a functional social system are greatly increased. In this chapter, I review the research literature regarding the relationship between poverty and family functioning. I draw a distinction between (a) stress from a simple drop in income or assets versus (b) a drop in income that puts the family economically below the poverty line. In particular, I examine the stress pileup from chronic poverty to better understand consequences—as well as alternative explanations—of this increasing U.S. family social stressor. First, concepts are defined and discussed. Then, theoretical explanations for understanding poverty in U.S. society are described. Following this, current empirical research is reviewed. The chapter concludes with discussion of gaps in the social work professional knowledge base and implications for practice.

CONCEPTS AND DEFINITIONS

In the midst of public controversy over poverty and welfare—and their "causes" and "consequences" for families—it is important to define a number of key concepts clearly, and understand them. Here, I delineate and briefly discuss the following terms: (a) poverty and poverty-line income, (b) relative poverty and absolute poverty, (c) working-poor families, (d) families on welfare, (e) family structure as it relates to poverty, and (f) families living in "urban ghettos."

Poverty and Poverty-Line Income

There are a number of complex issues in defining the often-used term *poverty*. Webster's dictionary (Gove, 1976) defines poverty in general as a "lack or relative lack of money or material possessions" or as being in a condition of "privation" or "want" (p. 1778). But there is no specification of what kinds or amounts of possessions are at issue—for example, basic necessities for food and shelter versus needing or wanting a variety of expensive consumer goods.

To address this ambiguity in the development of public policy, Mollie Orshansky and the U.S. Social Security Administration in 1964 developed an official "poverty-line" formula (for a detailed discussion, see Ozawa, 1982; see also Devine & Wright, 1993; Ruggles, 1990). Based on studies of the spending patterns of "poor" (i.e., low-income) families, Orshansky set a dollar price on an emergency monthly food budget, assuming that the "poverty" would be *temporary* (note also that this was based on a *minimally adequate* diet). After researchers in a 1955 study found that about one third of an average low-income family's monthly income was spent on food, the food budget was multiplied by three. Multiplying by 12 (months per year) provided an official annual "poverty line." Separate calculations were made for various sizes of households, assuming that two or more could live proportionately more cheaply than one. In addition, separate (lower) thresholds were calculated for farm families, based on the assumption that they could grow some of their own food.

This minimally adequate food budget multiplied by three, modified for family size—with annual adjustments based on the Consumer Price Index—has been used as a standard in the United States since 1964. The distinction between farm and nonfarm families has been eliminated. Separate thresholds are now calculated for Alaska and Hawaii. The 1995 federal poverty guidelines are shown in Figure 8.1. Thus, the poverty line for a family of four in the continental United States for 1995 is $15,150 (U.S. DHHS, 1995).

As can be seen from the above description, the fact that an individual or family has income at—or even slightly above—the poverty line does not ensure that the household has *adequate* income if adequate is

Household Size	Poverty Income Threshold*
1 person	$ 7,470
2 persons	10,030
3 persons	12,590
4 persons	15,150
5 persons	17,710
6 persons	20,270
7 persons	22,830
8 persons	25,390

Figure 8.1. 1995 U.S. Annual Poverty-Line Income for a Family of Four

SOURCE: U.S. Department of Health and Human Services (1995).
*Thresholds for Alaska and Hawaii are somewhat higher for each category.

defined as sufficient for stable, healthy living. It seems obvious that a food budget designed for a *minimally* adequate diet in an *emergency* and temporary situation is not sufficient for raising healthy children over the long term. It can also be argued that, especially with the rise in housing and utility costs over the past decade, the multiplier for the food budget should be raised from three to four—or even five—thereby pushing the poverty line to an even higher dollar amount (for further discussion of these baseline issues, see Devine & Wright, 1993).

As shown in Figure 8.2, a family of four attempting to live at or below the official poverty line would not have sufficient income in many U.S. communities to pay all the bills. As Rank (1994) illustrates in interviews with low-income households, often the family deals with the shortfall by juggling partial payments—one month, pay the rent, but make only a partial payment on the utilities; next month, reverse the pattern. This strategy can soon result in utility cutoffs and eviction, with no prospects for catching up.

It should be noted that the poverty line does not address the issue of assets, only of current income. This can make a difference in attempts to understand poverty and "adequacy." For example, a family that owns a home (an asset) in an area with relatively lower utilities, taxes, and repair costs may be far better off at a similar income level than a

Housing & Utilities	$ 422
Food & Household Supplies (@$28/person/week)	482
Clothing (@ $26/person/month)	104
Health Care (@$26/person/month)	104
Transportation (1 person, @$1.03 per day)	31
Laundry, Personal Items, Telephone, School Supplies, Work Supplies (@$1.00/person/day)	120
Monthly Total:	$1263
[Yearly Total (x 12):	$15, 150]

Figure 8.2. Monthly Poverty-Line "Budget" for a Family of Four (1995)

household that must rent housing in a relatively competitive market. Poverty policy in the United States does address the issue of assets by "means-testing" many income maintenance programs, such as AFDC. To establish eligibility for assistance, the household must "spend down" —that is, liquidate and live off of—any accumulated assets prior to receiving a grant. Any subsequent outside resources—such as an inheritance—must be reported and are then deducted from the grant amount. As a result, low-income families who find themselves needing assistance must often become and remain not only income poor but also asset poor (for a further discussion of this issue, see Sherraden, 1991). A few changes have recently been made in the spend-down requirements for some programs. For example, for an elderly couple applying for Medicaid, a home that they own and in which they currently reside can now be exempted from the asset means test. Some states are also experimenting with various kinds of asset limits and exemptions.

In the research I review here, such terms as *poverty, economic hardship, financial distress, economic deprivation,* and *economic strain* have often been operationalized in a variety of ways. Based on the above discussion, however, it can be logically argued that a study that categorizes families as "in poverty"—as operationalized by income that is at or below the federal poverty guidelines—is generally describing groups of households with income that is less than adequate to meet their minimum economic needs. Interestingly, at least one federal program for low-income families—the Women, Infants, and Children (WIC) program—uses income at or above *185% of the official poverty line* as the eligibility cutoff point for assistance (see Dolgoff et al., 1993, p. 223).

Relative Poverty and Absolute Poverty

The conceptualization and measurement of poverty described in the preceding section is referred to as an "absolute poverty" approach, contrasting with a "relative poverty" approach that has been used for a number of years by some researchers and in some other countries (Zimbalist, 1977). As discussed by a number of authors (e.g., Devine & Wright, 1993; Dolgoff et al., 1993; Ruggles, 1990; Schiller, 1989), if poverty and adequacy are delineated in terms of "resources needed to live comfortably and safely" (Devine & Wright, 1993, p. 2), "a decent standard . . . of well-being" (Gilbert, Specht, & Terrell, 1993, p. 58), or perhaps "a decent, frugal standard of living," then increases in the *general* population's standard of living must be taken into account in designating families and family members as "in poverty" versus "having enough." For example, if in today's society it is necessary to have a telephone to find work and a car to keep the job, it could be argued that these are now "basic necessities" for "a decent, frugal standard of living."

One way to measure relative poverty is to designate the bottom 20% (or lowest-income quintile) of the population as being in poverty. Solving the poverty problem then becomes impossible, as there will—by definition—always be a lowest-income quintile (Devine & Wright, 1993). Alternatively, some researchers argue for designating as in poverty any family that has "less than 50 percent of the median U.S. family income" (Dolgoff et al., 1993, p. 139). Dolgoff et al. also note, "Interestingly, at the time when Mollie Orshansky introduced the poverty measure for a four person family, the poverty level set forth was approximately one-half of the median income" (p. 139). In the 1990s, operationalizing the poverty line as a relative (50% of median income) versus absolute (minimally adequate food budget multiplied by three, modified for family size) threshold would add several thousand dollars to the current poverty line (p. 139). Although this would result in a currently perhaps politically unpalatable necessity to count additional large numbers of individuals and families as in poverty, social work and other human service professionals should advocate that such painful realities must no longer be hidden from view.

Working-Poor Families

As will be discussed further in a subsequent section on theoretical explanations, one of the myths associated with poor families in the United States is that poverty results from people's refusal to work, and therefore if adult family members would only get a job, the problem of poverty in the United States would be solved. As discussed in previous chapters, for increasing numbers of households it now takes at least two family providers to produce enough income for a decent standard of living. Ellwood (1988) concludes,

> Work does not always guarantee a route out of poverty. A full-time minimum-wage job . . . does not even come close to supporting a family of three at the poverty line. Even one full-time job and one half-time job at the minimum wage will not bring a family of four up to the poverty line. (p. 88)

In addition, "Half the poor children in America are living in two-parent homes" (p. 85); consequently, contrary to public perceptions, poverty is not confined to single-parent households. To be working in U.S. society today—whether full-time, full-year at minimum wages, or less than full-time (e.g., part-time or part-year in the secondary labor market, with alternating periods of employment and unemployment) even at slightly higher wages—does not preclude also living in poverty, particularly for a family with dependent children.

Families on Welfare

Like poverty, the term *welfare* in the United States today is often controversial and is also defined in a variety of ways. Sherraden (1991, pp. 60-69) argues convincingly that it is necessary to understand both "nonpoor welfare" programs (e.g., social security, including Medicare; tax subsidies for retirement pensions and home ownership, etc.) as well as the "poor welfare state" (i.e., welfare for the poor) or "targeted" welfare.

Current public debates regarding welfare and welfare reform often focus almost exclusively on the AFDC program. Other programs targeting individuals and families experiencing poverty include Supplemental

Security Income (SSI), general assistance (GA), food stamps, WIC (the Special Supplemental Food Program for Women, Infants, and Children), the Free or Reduced-Price School Lunch Program, Medicaid, and housing assistance programs (see Rank, 1994, pp. 22-24).

The term *families on welfare,* or *welfare families,* can be operationalized in a variety of ways—often depending on one's theoretical perspective (see subsequent sections). When used to designate families who are receiving AFDC benefits, the term certainly delineates a subset of families in poverty, as current benefit levels for AFDC fall below—and in some states dramatically below—current poverty guidelines (in Mississippi, in January 1992, the AFDC grant for a three-person family was $129 per month, or $1,548 per year; see Dolgoff et al., 1993, p. 199).

Family Structure and Poverty

As noted above, living in a two-parent family does not ensure escape from poverty. Nor are all one-parent households poor. Because of changes in economic structures discussed in Chapters 4 and 6, a family with only one wage earner—particularly when the wage earner is a woman—is increasingly likely to have income below the poverty line, however. If the single-parent female-headed household is without income (earned or otherwise) and is able to establish eligibility to receive a monthly AFDC benefit, the family will live below—or well below—the poverty line due to low benefit levels.

Thus, although family structure is not the only demographic factor associated with poverty (other factors include race, ethnicity, education, and whether there are children or other dependents in the household), "independent family households headed by a woman" face an increased likelihood of living in poverty (Ellwood, 1988, p. 129). In addition, "Poverty in single-parent families lasts much longer than it does in two-parent families" (p. 128).

Families Living in Urban Ghettos

In addition to emphasizing that subsets of both working and unemployed—two-parent and single-parent—families currently find themselves living in poverty, Ellwood (1988) describes a "small subset of poor families who live in the ghetto" (p. 190), defined as "a neighborhood with a poverty rate of 40 percent in a moderate-size or large city" (p. 193). Such families face

> a frightening array of negative forces: deprivation, concentration, isolation, discrimination, poor education, and the movement of jobs away from central cities. Add crime, drugs and alcohol, the underground economy, and welfare to these forces, and you have a combination of factors that would be hard for even the strongest and most concerned parents to fight. (p. 200)

Even so, not all people living in "high-poverty urban neighborhoods" (Ellwood, 1988, p. 195) are poor. In addition, many of the residents of such neighborhoods—whether poor or nonpoor—do not engage in such deviant behaviors as crime and drug use. Nor do all children drop out of school or become teenage parents. Overall, Ellwood (1988) emphasizes, "The full-time working poor, the retired and disabled, divorced mothers struggling to get on their feet, unemployed workers, rural farmers, young families who are starting out—these are much closer to the true faces of American poverty" (p. 194).

THEORETICAL EXPLANATIONS

Because delineations of the "cause(s)" of a particular problem are logically then often used to devise interventions to "solve" that problem —and also because causal theory building usually involves a particular set of assumptions or a specific paradigmatic worldview—the search for the cause(s), or theoretical explanations, of poverty has often been an intense and controversial enterprise. In a recent overview, Rank (1994) summarizes eight "explanations for poverty and welfare recipiency" (p. 25) and then proposes his own "structural vulnerability explanation" (p. 176), based on an extensive quantitative and qualitative empirical study of welfare recipients in Wisconsin. Using Rank's overview, I briefly delineate the following theoretical perspectives: (a) attitudinal or motivational explanations, (b) human capital explanations, (c) the culture of poverty, (d) the social isolation explanation, (e) Marxism, (f) dual labor market theory, (g) functionalism, (h) the Big Brother argument, and (i) structural vulnerability.

Attitudinal or Motivational Explanations

Attitudinal or motivational explanations posit that people are poor because of problematic individual motivations or attitudes, such as "lack of thrift, lack of effort, lack of ability and talent, and loose morals and drunkenness" (Rank, 1994, p. 26). Therefore, "provided they work hard enough," poor people will be able to escape poverty through individually changing these behaviors, attitudes, and motivations (p. 26). On the other hand, although such attitudes and motivations may at times be manifested by some poor people (as well as by some nonpoor people), it has been demonstrated empirically that the basic underlying assumption of this explanation—that there are stable jobs available at wages that will bring all individuals and families to "a decent, frugal standard of living"—is not tenable (see, e.g., Caputo, 1991; Ellwood, 1988). Until this assumption can be empirically demonstrated as having been met, this perspective must be viewed with skepticism as perhaps a partial description of some people (whether poor or nonpoor) at certain times in their lives—but an inadequate explanation of poverty.

Human Capital Explanations

Also focusing on the individual person, the human capital perspective posits that in order to reduce poverty, individuals must acquire "additional training, education, experience, skills, and so on" (Rank, 1996, p. 27). It is argued that these additional personal resources, by increasing individuals' stores of "human capital," will enable these persons to compete more effectively in the labor market and thus to escape poverty (Rank, 1994, pp. 26-27). Like the previous explanation, however, this perspective is based on a currently untenable assumption that if these individuals expand their human capital, there will be jobs available at wages that will provide a decent, frugal standard of living for themselves and their families. Until this assumption can be met, simply providing or requiring further training may only end in frustration and disillusionment for many of the poor persons and families who are being advised or mandated to work their way out of poverty.

The Culture of Poverty

The culture of poverty perspective shifts from a strictly individual focus to an emphasis on community "culture," or sets of group beliefs, values, and norms. According to this view, poverty becomes "part of a cultural process in which children learn from their parents and from their surrounding environment that relying on public assistance, bearing children out of wedlock, dropping out of school, and so on, are acceptable behaviors" (Rank, 1994, p. 28). Although the description of behaviors reflected in this perspective may be at least partially accurate for some families in some urban ghetto neighborhoods, the theoretical explanation does not address whether such behaviors—where they exist—are the *cause(s)* of poverty versus the *consequence(s)* of poverty. If such beliefs are adaptations to conditions of economic deprivation and consequent social disorganization, then changes in community beliefs *and* economic conditions must occur in relation to each another. Thus, over the long term, the key component may be not specific beliefs but stable economic development.

The Social Isolation Explanation

The social isolation explanation is focused specifically on poverty in urban ghetto neighborhoods, based on extensive studies of such communities in Chicago by William Julius Wilson (1987). In Rank's (1994) summary, "As the black middle and working classes have left the inner cities, fewer positive role models are present in the community. The inner city has become more socially isolated, while at the same time experiencing a greater concentration of deviant behavior" (p. 29). Such a view does posit that "A distinct culture exists in the inner city" (p. 30), but it rests on the assumption that "The ultimate cause of inner-city conditions is not the culture itself but the social structural constraints and the lack of opportunities" (p. 29).

Thus, the social isolation argument is linked to at least some of the theoretical explanations focused on larger social systems. These perspectives emphasize structural factors to explain poverty and to address the problems associated with being poor. As Ellwood (1988) points out in his discussion of urban ghetto poverty, however, people who are experiencing poverty and social isolation in inner-city neighborhoods represent only a small subset of individuals and families in poverty in the United States today.

Marxism

As Rank (1994) notes, "Marxism focuses on the economic structure of capitalism as the key to understanding poverty" (p. 30). He goes on to explain, "According to Marx, then, poverty is simply inherent in the economic structure of capitalism—it is an inevitable by-product of the exploitation of workers by capitalists. To eradicate poverty, one must change the entire capitalist system" (p. 31). The specific social structures projected to be demonstrably effective in eradicating poverty in a new system are not as clearly articulated—resulting in a clear critique of the old system but fairly vague recommendations for new economic structures.

Dual Labor Market Theory

As discussed in Chapter 6, dual labor market theory describes

> Two quite distinct markets that operate according to different rules. In the primary market, jobs are characterized by stability, high wages, good working conditions, a greater degree of internal job structure, and unionization. . . . On the other hand, jobs in the secondary labor market are characterized as menial, having poor working conditions, and low wages. (Rank, 1994, p. 31)

In this view, Rank notes,

> People are poor not because they are unemployed or do not participate in the economy but because of the way in which they participate in the economy. Because of the instability of jobs in the secondary labor market, workers in them often experience occasional unemployment and turn to welfare programs in order to survive lean times. (p. 32)

In addition, "Employers in the primary labor market...use these [unstable work histories of workers from the secondary labor market] as evidence that they are inadequate workers, and thus they are blocked from moving into the primary market" (p. 32). In this view, then, expanding the number of jobs in the primary labor market; providing expanded opportunities for movement into those jobs; and ensuring adequate employment, wages, and income for workers in the secondary labor market would all be potential avenues for beginning to address the problem of poverty.

Functionalism

A third structural explanation of poverty is functionalism, which, Rank (1994) argues, posits that

> Poverty serves a number of important functions for society in general and specifically . . . it serves important economic, social, cultural, and political functions for the affluent class. (p. 33)

For example, the existence of poverty ensures that undesirable work gets done and creates a number of occupations and professions serving the poor (e.g., academics writing books about the poor); the poor can be identified and punished as deviants in order to uphold the legitimacy of dominant norms; and so on. (p. 33)

Thus, "Phenomena like poverty can be eliminated only when they either become sufficiently dysfunctional for the affluent or when the poor can obtain enough power to change the system of social stratification" (Gans, cited in Rank, 1994, p. 33). Perhaps because of its level of abstraction, this view often seems based on the assumption of some kind of "invisible [functional] hand" that somehow automatically brings about change in current social systems, systems that appear to deterministically "function" beyond or in spite of personal human actions and constructions.

The Big Brother Argument

The Big Brother argument is focused particularly on welfare use, as follows:

> Human nature is characterized as desiring the easiest way out of difficult situations. In the case of poverty, welfare and charity create work disincentives. Individuals exert themselves less when in dire straits because they know they can fall back on the safety net of public assistance. As they become more accustomed to receiving welfare, they eventually settle into the lifestyle. (Rank, 1994, p. 34)

Thus,

> From this point of view, the solution to the problem of poverty is to cut back substantially on social welfare programs and to ensure that work disincentives are minimized in the remaining programs. Governmental intrusion into private initiative must be curtailed so that people have no choice but to work themselves out of poverty. (p. 35)

Although, according to this perspective, structural incentives and disincentives may be important in understanding and addressing poverty issues, it also relies on the untenable assumption, as discussed above, that it is currently possible for poor people in the United States to work themselves out of poverty.

A Structural Vulnerability Explanation

Based on data from a longitudinal caseload sample of welfare recipients in Wisconsin, in-depth qualitative interviews with a random sample of those recipients in one representative county, and field observations and interviews in the Wisconsin welfare system and the sampled community, Rank (1994) proposes "a structural vulnerability explanation" that he argues can assist in understanding "how the various pieces of the [poverty and welfare] puzzle fit together" (p. 176). This theoretical perspective is based on a multilevel approach in that it "combines aspects of human capital theory with the more structural components of our society" (p. 176)—thus focusing both on the individual and on larger social systems. Using the musical chairs metaphor (described and discussed in Chapter 6), Rank notes that, although the "losers" in the employment and unemployment (and related poverty and adequacy) competition "will generally be those who lack human capital and thus cannot compete as effectively as those who have acquired greater human capital" (p. 184), nevertheless "we should not mistake an analysis of the losers for an analysis of the game itself" (Wright & Lam, cited p. 184). In summary, Rank argues,

> People lacking human capital are more economically vulnerable if a crisis occurs. Such crises are often the result of broader economic, social, and political forces in our society. In addition, the lack of human capital is largely a result of the reproduction of social class. Children from lower-class backgrounds begin with fewer resources and opportunities, which in turn limits their future life chances and outcomes, including the accumulation of human capital. Finally, although lack of human capital and the vulnerability this leads to explain who the losers of the economic game are, the more structural components of our economic, social, and political systems explain why there are losers in the first place. (p. 185)

Although in his discussions Rank (1994) seems to focus primarily on two levels, (a) the person and (b) social structures at more macro social systems levels, his approach can theoretically encompass all seven systems levels delineated in Chapter 2 (person, family, neighborhood, local community, state, nation, and globe). Rank also discusses some possible neighborhood and community-level—in addition to individual and structural—interventions to address poverty issues (pp. 194-196). Given his attention to low-income workers' and their families' vulnerability to economic and social crises—especially because of low wages, limited resources, and recurring periods of unemployment—the stress and coping framework appears quite compatible with Rank's structural vulnerability theoretical perspective, both for understanding poverty and for devising, implementing, and evaluating potentially effective multilevel interventions.

RESEARCH FINDINGS

As a way of organizing the empirical literature on poverty and its relationship to families, I discuss findings from recent research under the following headings: (a) current statistics and longitudinal trends, (b) correlates and consequences of poverty, and (c) poverty programs and their evaluation.

Statistics and Trends

To work effectively with families—and in policy and advocacy roles —social workers need (a) accurate descriptions of current societal *reality,* (b) an understanding of poverty and inequality *trends* over the past several decades, and (c) an understanding of *populations* that are particularly at risk for poverty and resulting difficulties.

Reality. Devine and Wright (1993) point out, "From 1983 through to the end of the decade, . . . nearly 35 million Americans lived at or below the official poverty standard each year" (p. 29). They go on to state,

> It is hard to appreciate just how large a number 35 million is. The number of the poor in the United States, for example, is approximately equal to the total combined population of the nation's forty largest cities, is larger than the population of Canada (by about ten million), and is twice the combined populations of the seven nations of Central America. There are four times more poor people than there are college students, six times more poor people than Jewish people, twenty times more poor people than there are writers, artists, entertainers, and athletes combined. There are more poor people in the United States than there are seconds in a year. (pp. 29-30)

Equally dramatic is discussion by Ruggles (1990) that if an alternative threshold is used, "calculated using the same general methods as the original Orshansky standard, but with a 'multiplier' updated to reflect the changing share of food in family budgets" (p. 55), then the 1987 poverty rate in the U.S. would have been 25.9%, or over *60 million* persons. Thus, in contrast with some public perceptions that the United States is a primarily middle-class nation—with only a small number of families living in or near poverty—the current societal reality in the national social system is that very large numbers of individuals and families are experiencing economic hardship and distress.

Trends. For some politicians and policymakers, the reality sketched above may seem an overwhelming and impossible problem, incapable of being "solved" and therefore better left more or less invisible. Studies of trends in poverty and inequality in the United States over the past several decades have found evidence that poverty can be addressed, however—at least to some extent—with certain kinds of policies and programs. For example, Zimmerman and Chilman (1988) note, "Poverty rates among the elderly have declined dramatically in recent years. . . . Such progress is largely due to expanded Social Security coverage and increased Social Security and Supplemental Security benefits for the elderly" (p. 111; see also Danziger, Sandefur, & Weinberg, 1994).

In addition, as depicted in Figure 8.3, Devine and Wright (1993) demonstrate that overall, "The number of the poor declined steadily throughout the 1960s, from 40 million poor at the beginning of the decade to about 25 million poor at the end" (p. 28). They also note, "The sharpest declines occurred after the onset of the War on Poverty in 1964" (p. 28), leading them to conclude that—contrary to the argument by some critics that the United States "lost" the War on Poverty—"We surrendered just as the tide was beginning to turn" (p. 31).

During the 1970s, the number of people in poverty fluctuated around 25 million. Between 1983 and 1989, with the Reagan administration's policies of (a) tax cuts for the wealthy and (b) reductions in social programs for the poor or near-poor—in combination with the macroeconomic changes in employment and wages discussed in Chapters 4 and 6—"the richest one-half of 1 percent of U.S. families received 55 percent of the total increase in household wealth while the bottom 60 percent of families found their wealth either stagnating or falling during that same period" (Schwartz & Scott, 1994, p. 434). During this time period, the number of poor people remained high (see Figure 8.3).

Populations at Risk. In the U.S. national system, some populations are more at risk of experiencing poverty than others. Schwartz and Scott

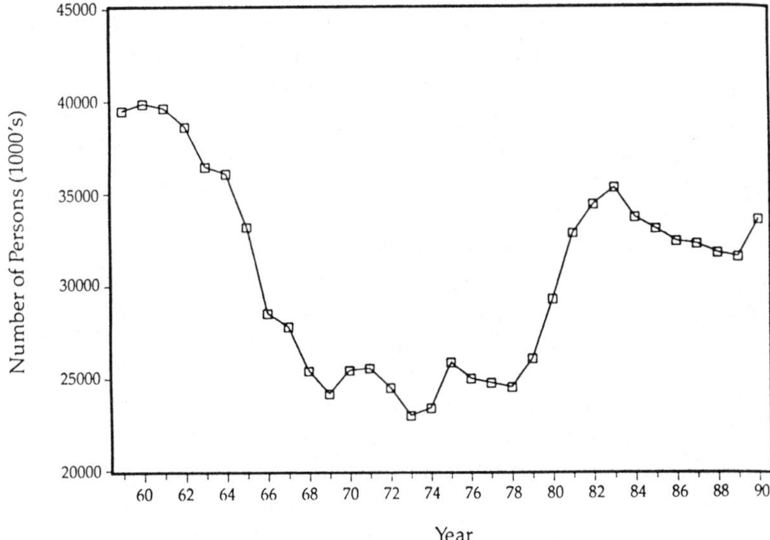

Figure 8.3. Number of Persons Below the Official Poverty Line, 1959-1990 (in thousands)

SOURCE: Devine and Wright (1993). Reprinted with permission from: Devine, Joel A. and Wright, James D. *The Greatest of Evils: Urban Poverty and the American Underclass.* (New York: Aldine de Gruyter) Copyright © 1993, Walter de Gruyter, Inc., New York.

(1994) note, "Families with children, families of color, families headed by women, and the unmarried elderly are especially vulnerable" (p. 434-435; see also Devine & Wright, 1993; Levy & Michel, 1991; Winnick, 1988; Zimmerman & Chilman, 1988). Such vulnerability is the result of a number of structural changes in the U.S. economic system. These include "the loss of high-paying jobs; the stagnation of wages; the growth of part-time and temporary employment; increased individual, business, and national debt; and a changed tax structure that shifted some tax burdens from businesses to individuals and from the wealthy to the middle class" (Schwartz & Scott, 1994, p. 435).

Of particular concern is the increasing number of children in the United States who are living in poverty (Devine & Wright, 1993; Segal, 1991; Winnick, 1988; Zimmerman & Chilman, 1988). Zimmerman and Chilman (1988) find, "The percentage of children aged 18 and under who were poor rose from 14% in 1969 to a disturbing 22% of the child population by 1984. This includes 18% of all white children and almost half of all black children. The highest poverty rates were for black and Hispanic children under age 6" (p. 110). In addition, they note that about a third of children in poverty "lived in persistently poor families"—that is, in families remaining in poverty for more than 4 years (p. 110). These authors found that in the mid-1980s, "The average black child is poor for 5 years of his or her life compared to 10 months for the average white child" (pp. 110-111).

In looking at poor people in the United States as a group, Devine and Wright (1993) note, "Just over half of the poor (50.8%) are outside the prime labor force participation ages, that is, are less than 18 [i.e., are children or youth] or more than 65 [i.e., are elderly]" (p. 50). In addition, "Almost 6 million poor Americans in 1990 lived in families where someone worked full time all year round. Here the major problem is not insufficient hours [of work] but inadequate wages" (p. 50). Thus, as noted above in the discussion of theoretical explanations of poverty, understandings that focus on attitudinal, motivational, cultural, or even human capital "causes" of poverty—and a strategy of programs that rely on the poor working themselves out of poverty—cannot be expected to be effective without at least concomitant understandings and strategies that address structural economic changes. These include opportunities for stable employment, adequate wages for families, and programs to ensure sufficient income for those not expected to work—including the elderly.

Correlates and Consequences

In light of large and increasing numbers of persons in the U.S. national social system experiencing the reality of poverty, it is important to understand correlates and consequences of being poor—and in particular how economic hardship affects families as well as individual family members. Here, I review six interrelated areas of empirical research findings: (a) housing, (b) physical health, (c) mental health, (d) parenting, (e) family relationships, and (f) family formation and dissolution.

Housing. Devine and Wright (1993) note, "The incidence of homelessness grew throughout the 1980s . . . in close tandem with the increasing poverty rate and especially with the increasing chronicity of poverty" (p. 118). They also note that homelessness imposes additional stresses in addition to the stress of chronic poverty. Newman (1993, p. 53) comments on the "impact of rising housing costs and stagnating paychecks." She states,

> Young people face steep increases in the cost of rents, up 28 percent since 1982. If wages had kept up with rents, this would not be a problem, but workers aged twenty-five to thirty-four were earning only 77 percent of the wages earned by people ten years older than themselves, down from 86 percent in 1980. (p. 53)

The impact of these trends—increasing poverty and increasing difficulties in finding affordable housing, including the experience of homelessness—are illuminated further by Mulroy (1990) in her study of families applying to participate in the federally funded Section 8 rental assistance program. She states, "Federal cutbacks in affordable housing programs during the Reagan years and a reduced supply of affordable rental units in the private market have created a housing crisis that is injurious to households headed by single mothers" (p. 542).

Some of the families she studied—people who could not be served by the rental assistance program because of funding limits—were doubling up with relatives. Others "lived in public housing projects they wanted to escape. Others lived in substandard units in the private rental market that landlords either refused to repair or tried to repair to a level below minimum housing quality standards" (p. 544). Although few studies have been focused directly on families in relationship to changes in housing patterns and policies over the past several decades, it seems clear that poverty puts families at risk for facing additional problems with access to adequate and stable housing—and that severe chronic poverty can result in a family experiencing the catastrophic stress of homelessness.

Physical Health. Zimmerman and Chilman (1988), in a review of findings on families and poverty, note that poverty has deleterious effects on the health of family members. Particularly striking is the fact that "Studies continue to show that poverty is a critical factor in infant mortality" (p. 119). These authors also call attention to the fact that "Poverty and ill health have been shown to have a debilitating reciprocal relationship. Poor people get sick because they are poor, and then because they are sick, they work less or lose their jobs and become poorer still" (pp. 119-120). In addition, severe budget cuts in federal funding for health care programs—for example, Medicaid and community health centers—has resulted in many families' having reduced access to adequate health care compared to a decade ago, including preventive services as well as treatment (Zimmerman & Chilman, 1988).

Mental Health. In the unemployment literature reviewed in Chapter 6, economic or financial hardship (also referred to as economic deprivation) has been identified as a stressor commonly associated with both poor health and poor mental health (Ferman & Gardner, 1979; Kessler et al., 1987, 1988; Ross, Mirowsky, & Goldsteen, 1990; Voydanoff, 1991).

Chilman (1991), in her review of the literature on working poor families, found "Economic hardship through unemployment or low wages reveal such psychological effects on both men and women as feelings of inferiority, inadequacy, depression, and frustration" (p. 192). In a review focused on black families, McLoyd (1990) notes, "Adults who are poor have more mental health problems than their economically advantaged counterparts" (p. 318). She goes on to state,

> Among the etiological factors responsible for the elevation of mental health problems among the poor is an overrepresentation in lower-class life of a broad range of frustration-producing life events and chronic conditions outside personal control. . . . Individuals who are poor are confronted with an unremitting succession of negative life events (e.g., eviction, physical illness, criminal assault) in the context of chronically stressful, ongoing life conditions such as inadequate housing and dangerous neighborhoods that together increase the exigencies of day-to-day existence. (p. 318)

Similarly, in recent studies of families negatively affected by the rural farm crisis in the United States, economic pressure and financial strain were associated with such stress reactions as hostility, withdrawal, and depression in both men and women (Armstrong & Schulman, 1990; Conger & Elder, 1994; Van Hook, 1990; see also Conger et al., 1991, 1992; Elder, Conger, Foster, & Ardelt, 1992; Whitbeck et al., 1991). Armstrong and Schulman (1990) found that a sense of "personal control" was also important in understanding the relationship between economic hardship and depression—that is, "The ability of farm operators to meet basic household needs has important [positive] consequences for their sense of control and emotional well-being" (p. 487).

Related to these findings, Thoits (1983, p. 85) has posited that decreases in sense of mastery and self-esteem—stemming from a pileup of stressful life events—may contribute to a "complex vicious cycle" of increasing psychological distress. Further, Ross et al. (1990; see also Mirowsky & Ross, 1989), in a review of relationships between economic and employment factors, family variables, and health, identify "the sense of not being in control of one's own life" as potentially diminishing "the will and motivation to actively solve problems. . . . "Little suc- cess [in solving life's problems, such as adequate income] over long periods discourages and demoralizes people, reinforcing the sense of powerlessness and fatalism" (p. 1073).

Parenting. Several important recent studies have documented a relationship between economic hardship—including poverty—and harsh or authoritarian parenting. Chilman (1991) reports that working-poor single mothers experiencing severe role overload "may be so stressed that at least some of them develop negative rejecting attitudes toward their young children" (p. 193).

Among two-parent farm and nonfarm families in Iowa, Conger and Elder (1994; in collaboration with Lorenz, Simons, Whitbeck, and others) found that economic pressure in the family—related to low family income, unstable work, an unfavorable debt-to-assets ratio, and income loss (see p. 10 and pp. 100-101)—predicted a parent's harsh and inconsistent disciplinary practices. Associations were both direct (in families with low spouse support) and indirect (through the parent's hostility toward the spouse) (p. 218). They also note, "In particular, children from displaced [farm] families were most likely to have fathers who were depressed and ineffective in problem solving, and consequently unlikely to assume a nurturing role as a parent. The children of these men scored relatively high on felt rejection by parents and on emotional distress" (p. 101; see also Conger et al., 1991, 1992; Whitbeck et al., 1991).

In a study of single mothers, Simons, Beaman, Conger, and Chao (1993) found that although economic pressure did not directly predict ineffective discipline (including harsh disciplinary practices, little behavioral monitoring, inconsistency in discipline, and failure to set clear standards), it did indirectly predict discipline through (a) number of negative life events (e.g., changing residence, death of a friend, getting robbed, having an automobile accident), and (b) psychological distress of the mother (depression and hostility). Similarly, McLoyd and Wilson (1990) found that for single mothers,

> While the level of economic hardship was unrelated to the child's psychological functioning, it was positively related to psychological distress in the mother. Psychological distress in the mother was positively related to psychological problems in the child. This pattern of findings is consistent with evidence suggesting that economic hardship, rather than having direct effects, adversely affects children's socioemotional functioning in part through its impact on the parent. (p. 65; see also Bank, Forgatch, Patterson, & Fetrow, 1993; Elder & Caspi, 1988)

In addition, McLoyd (1990) concludes, "Child abuse represents an extreme form of punitive parenting that occurs more frequently in families experiencing economic decline than in families with stable resources" (p. 324). She elaborates:

> Existing research supports the conclusion that poverty and economic loss generally result in more punitive and less nurturant, supportive behavior by parents, especially if their children are temperamentally difficult and physically unattractive. This conclusion is buttressed by research on child abuse. The relation between economic hardship and punitive, inconsistent parenting behavior seems to stem from increased levels of anxiety, irritability, and depression experienced by economically deprived parents. (p. 327)

Family Relationships. In addition to influencing parent-child relationships, economic hardship and financial distress have been shown to affect other family relationships as well—including marital and sibling relationships. Voydanoff and Donnelly (1988) found that overall economic distress (including economic deprivation, economic strain, employment instability, and employment uncertainty) was negatively related to marital and family satisfaction. Conger et al. (1990) found, "Economic pressures had an indirect association with married couples' evaluation of the marriage by promoting hostility in marital interactions and curtailing the warm and supportive behaviors spouses express toward one another" (p. 643; see also Conger & Elder, 1994). Similarly, Johnson and Booth (1990) found that economic distress "had clear [negative] effects on marital quality of farm couples. . . . Farmers undergoing financial distress showed a substantial increase over the 5 years of the study in their likelihood of entertaining thoughts of divorce" (p. 164).

Conger et al. (1992) found that economic hardship—through father's and mother's depressed mood—predicted higher marital conflict (p. 535); lower marital conflict predicted more nurturant and involved parenting by each parent—resulting in male seventh-grade children's more positive adjustment (pp. 536-537). In addition, Conger and Elder (1994) found that mother's and father's hostility increased hostility between siblings (pp. 249-250); they note, "Siblings may emulate their parents' hostile interactional style in their own interactions" and, "Of particular interest was the strong negative effect parents' hostility had on warm and supportive feelings between siblings" (p. 251). They conclude,

> Taken together, the results . . . suggest that the economic decline experienced by Iowa families during the 1980s had a significant and lasting impact on their emotional well-being and interpersonal relations. Today, many of these families have become chronically stressed by their economic circumstances. . . . Financial difficulties directly increase risk for emotional problems, especially among parents. Personal unhappiness and irritability translate into hostile and angry behaviors with other family members, including children. The data show that these disrupted patterns of behavior threaten the perceived quality of family relationships for all family members. Ultimately, family conflict and turmoil increases the risk of adjustment problems in the developmental trajectories of children and adolescents. (pp. 263-264)

Family Formation and Dissolution. In a review of relationships between economic hardship, marital bonds, and mental health, McLoyd (1990) concludes, "Economic hardship promotes marital dissolution and deters marriage among couples who have children and those who do not" (p. 319). Similarly, Zimmerman and Chilman (1988) note,

> The potential consequences of poverty, especially long-term and severe poverty, are serious in many ways. For instance, through adapting to its corrosive effects, individuals and families may develop feelings of hopelessness, distrust, despair, fear, hostility, and fatalism. . . . [Such] attitudes and feelings . . . can impede the development of positive, committed marital relationships and erode existing marriages, especially when they are combined with environmental conditions characterized by high unemployment, poor housing, hunger, neighborhood disorganization, poor health, and the absence of money. (pp. 120-121)

In summary, poverty often involves a pileup of multiple stresses that together can destabilize families. As Chilman (1991) points out, "Family poverty . . . is strongly correlated with high rates of school-age childbearing, school failure, violent crimes, bad health in infancy and childhood, malnutrition, child abuse and neglect, and lack of access to social and health services. . . . Long-term severe poverty tends to have particularly adverse effects on child and family development. (p. 193)

Programs and Evaluation

Given the potentially catastrophic picture of stress pileup for many low-income families—particularly families experiencing severe or chronic poverty—it is important to understand procedural knowledge from current research findings regarding the effectiveness of programs that have already been designed to address these problems and stressors. First, I delineate overall U.S. strategies and compare them to alternatives in other Western industrial societies. Next, I briefly review findings from recent evaluations of specific welfare reform programs. Finally, I identify several policies with impacts that have not yet been thoroughly evaluated.

Strategies. A number of authors over the years have commented on the lack of overall poverty and family policies in the U.S. system of social welfare (see, e.g., Kamerman & Kahn, 1981; Rodgers, 1990). In Rodgers's (1990) summary:

> The social welfare systems of other major Western industrial societies differ from the American system in several important respects. First, most of these countries provide a broader core of universal, non-means-tested assistance programs to all citizens. The most obvious example is the package of programs provided to all citizens through the health-care system. Second, the countries have programs specifically designed to assist families with children. These programs are either universal or provided to almost all middle- and low-income families. All the countries make this package available to lone-parent families, with many giving such families a larger supplement. Third, none of them denies assistance to intact families or requires a lone parent to stay unemployed, single, or poor to qualify for, or remain qualified for, critical assistance such as housing or health care. Fourth, the cash-benefit programs are uniform for all poor families, regardless of family structure. (pp. 115-116)

These differences in programs and policies can be understood from a social systems perspective as being embedded in differing national beliefs (explanations) about poverty and its causes. In the United States, values of individualism and the work ethic have resulted in a tendency to focus on individual-level "causes" or explanations of poverty, often ignoring structural factors and understandings. In spite of numerous recent studies of labor market changes in the U.S. national economic system and the impacts of poverty on families and family members, many politicians and voting citizens continue to believe that poverty can be solved by individuals' simply getting a job and working their way out of poverty.

As a result, strategies and programs to address poverty and its consequences in the United States continue to be fragmented—and subject to reduced funding in an era of budget cuts and "no new taxes" (Danziger et al., 1994). Policies that partially address certain needs of some low-income families in the United States are the often-controversial welfare programs AFDC, Medicaid, food stamps, housing assistance, general assistance, the school lunch program, SSI, WIC, and so forth. (Rank, 1994). In addition, some family members may qualify for less-controversial social security benefits (retired workers, disabled workers, or survivors of a deceased worker). Some families now benefit from the Earned Income Tax Credit (EITC). Many low-income families disrupted by stress are served by the child welfare system, but these services are often focused primarily on the child or the family as a social system and unable to address effectively chronic income deprivation and neighborhood disorganization in inner-city ghetto communities (see, e.g., Dore, 1993; Nelson, Saunders, & Landsman, 1993).

Evaluation of Welfare Reform Programs. Controversy over the AFDC program has led to a variety of state and local initiatives to reform welfare, a number of which have been carefully empirically evaluated. In an overview and summary of studies by the Manpower Demonstration Research Corporation, Gueron and Pauly (1991) conclude that aspects of recent welfare-to-work programs were successful with some households: "Overall, they increased the earnings of poor families and saved money. However, they did not eliminate welfare or poverty" (p. ix).

Similarly, Levitan and Gallo (1993), in an evaluation of the Job Opportunities and Basic Skills (JOBS) component of the 1988 Family

Support Act, note, "The most serious deficiency of JOBS is its failure to create jobs for recipients unable to find work in the regular economy" (p. iv). In addition, they conclude, "The problems of welfare are closely intertwined with poverty, and the two should be addressed in concert. Policymakers have too long ignored the fact that genuine welfare reform is impossible without addressing the needs of the working poor" (p. v).

Policies Needing Further Evaluation. As Devine and Wright (1993) point out, there is considerable controversy over whether the 1960s War on Poverty was "beginning to win" or "lost" (p. 31). Different retrospective methods of study and theoretical perspectives result in varying conclusions. National studies of social security indicate that this program has been reasonably successful in alleviating poverty among many of the elderly in the United States, although some elderly persons—particularly women—continue to experience poverty (Devine & Wright, 1993; Ozawa, 1982).

Newman (1993) suggests that following World War II, low-interest mortgages and the GI Bill were effective in supporting education and home ownership, especially among young families of returning servicemen. Thus, she argues, contrary to the "hard work" and "pull yourself up by your own bootstraps" view of achievement among many from that generation, "The hard work paid off only because economic conditions over which no individual had control made it possible and because government policies provided a helping hand" (pp. 221-222).

Other programs needing further study in the context of the national social system are the 1930s and 1940s WPA and other national recovery programs, impacts of changes in the minimum wage (e.g., Mincy, 1990), and understandings of effects from newer programs and proposals, such as the EITC, refundable child care credits, and asset accumulation policies (Sherraden, 1991).

KNOWLEDGE GAPS

As indicated in Figure 8.4, especially in an urban ghetto neighborhood, to attempt to address only family issues—or only one larger-system issue (e.g., education or jobs or crime or mental health) at a time—is likely to result in frustration for practitioners at direct service and program and policy levels as well as for families and neighborhood organizations. Seeing families and neighborhoods from a social systems

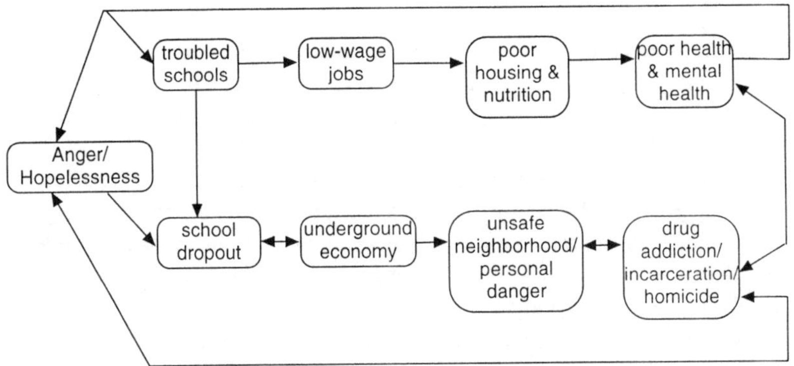

Figure 8.4. Multiple Stressors Associated With Poverty in an Urban Ghetto Neighborhood

perspective may begin to assist with the development and evaluation of more effective strategies and programs for addressing the complex and interactive problems of poverty.

Thus, based on a developmental social systems stress and coping perspective, further knowledge building is essential at multiple systems levels if the catastrophic legacies of stress pileup from poverty among U.S. families is to be alleviated or prevented. At the family system level, understandings are needed regarding effective ways of restabilizing families and how much time restabilization requires. A social systems perspective would suggest that restabilization of a *previously stable* family would be very different—and would likely take considerably less time—than stabilization of a *chronically stressed* family that has experienced crisis after crisis, leaving family members throughout the extended-family system exhausted from recurrent overwhelming changes. A social systems framework would also suggest that effective work with a family living in a *stable neighborhood*—where a majority of households have access, at a minimum, to a stable, frugal, decent standard of living—is very different, in both time frame and methods, from work with a family living in a disorganized and dangerous *urban ghetto,* where a majority of households may live in increasingly severe and chronic poverty and where daily living is often a struggle for survival.

Effective methods for social work practice at macro levels are also critical. Community development models and methods for various kinds of city neighborhoods, small towns, and rural areas must continue to be developed, evaluated, and disseminated. Similarly, effective local and state programs and policies for economic development and for addressing poverty and other related social needs are essential.

At the national and international levels, continuing efforts are needed in understanding social systems as complex interactive entities. Within and among social systems levels, economic structures and policies, political roles and structures, and a variety of beliefs and ideologies (influenced by the media) affect how citizens and policymakers understand poverty as well as what changes in policies and programs are feasible and under what conditions.

As discussed in Chapter 1, development of both propositional and procedural knowledge requires a continuing process of developing theoretical explanations and hypotheses, empirically testing hypotheses, and drawing conclusions from the findings to refine and further develop theories and models. Such knowledge building efforts are vitally needed at multiple levels to address causes, consequences, and effective solutions for poverty.

SUMMARY

In summary, a variety of theoretical explanations for poverty have been developed, many of which require further empirical testing. Much empirical research has been done, although some has been atheoretical and therefore in need of further development into usable theories and models. Current findings, developed in large part from social systems, structural vulnerability, and stress and coping theoretical approaches, include:

1. Poverty is a reality for many families and has increased in the United States over the past decade, particularly among women, children and people of color.
2. Poverty is associated with unstable housing and homelessness. Stress pileup—found especially in association with *chronic* poverty—can result in deleterious outcomes for family members' physical and mental health, as well as problems in parent-child and other family relationships. In addition, studies suggest that poverty can delay or inhibit family formation. Chronic poverty and associated stress pileup can also result in marital instability and family dissolution.

3. Evaluations of policies and programs to address poverty yield findings that programs focused primarily on the individual or the family are often ineffective in addressing problems connected with larger-system functioning, such as low wages; lack of benefits (e.g., health care coverage); unemployment; and lack of stable, affordable support services at neighborhood and community levels.

As will be discussed in detail in the next chapter, at both micro and macro levels, social work practitioners and researchers are needed who are committed over the long term to working together to develop empirically based professional knowledge regarding: (a) how families are affected by stress from increasing poverty; (b) comprehensive understandings of societal *costs* of *not* effectively addressing family poverty; (c) what kinds of interventions are—and are not—effective at specific social systems levels for particular problems and populations; and (d) what policies and programs, at agency, neighborhood, local, state, national, and international levels, are effective in addressing poverty and its associated stressors for families and family members.

It is clear that within the U.S. national social system, it is possible to grow enough food; build adequate shelter; and train teachers, health care workers, and other human service professionals to ensure a decent, frugal standard of living for all individuals and families. Specifics regarding models, methods, time tables, and so on for how—over time—to develop social systems that make that goal a reality are currently not at all clear. For me, at least, participating in the continuing struggle to meet that challenge is a life work that is well worth doing.

Chapter 9

FAMILIES AND POVERTY
Applications and Tools for Practice

CASE SCENARIO

The genogram in Figure 9.1 shows the Jones family at a time of major transition. Tanya, age 20, has been raised by her maternal grandparents because of her mother's heroin addiction. She completed high school and has been working for minimum wage at a fast-food restaurant. She has been seeing Dennis for nearly a year, and they have discussed marriage on several occasions. He has not been able to find stable work, however and was recently charged with drug possession. Tanya is now pregnant, and the family is encouraging her not to have an abortion. Both she and Dennis would like to establish a household of their own, but her wages, even supplemented by his day laborer's wages, are not enough to cover rent and other basic necessities for a new family. Tanya's grandmother, Rose, has recently been diagnosed with cancer and is unsure whether she would be able to care for a new great-grandchild. Her grandfather, Leroy, has emphysema and receives an SSI benefit. He has recently been staying with a relative, saying that he "can't stand the confusion" of Rose and Tanya arguing about what to do about Tanya's pregnancy.

Scenario 1

Figure 9.2 shows one possible scenario for the Jones family in their efforts to cope with Tanya and Dennis's transition to parenthood, following the birth of Michael. In September, 2 weeks after Michael's birth, Dennis and Tanya moved into an apartment with some "borrowed" financial assistance from Leroy. By December, they were behind on both rent and

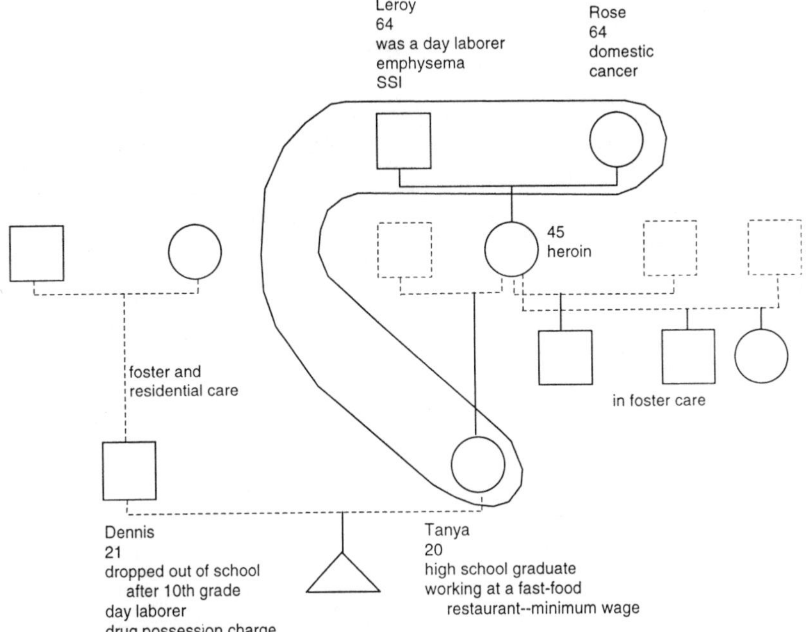

Figure 9.1. Jones Family Genogram

utilities, and Dennis began helping a "friend" transport drugs—to "try to help pay the bills"—and anxiety and conflict between Dennis and Tanya escalated. In January, after an argument in which Dennis slapped Tanya and stormed out of the apartment, Tanya packed and moved with Michael back to her grandmother's home.

Rose was upset about Dennis's continuing involvement with drugs and continually criticized Tanya for leaving Michael with a friend (who was also a young mother) while she worked at the fast-food restaurant. By April, Rose and Tanya's relationship was alternating between active arguing and yelling, or hostilely "ignoring" one another. In May, Dennis promised that he would change his ways. After borrowing a month's rent from a friend, he persuaded Tanya to move with Michael into a new apartment with him.

During the summer, Tanya continued to work, often leaving Michael with Dennis, especially when she worked the night shift. Dennis was unable to find a stable job, and arguing between Dennis and Tanya escalated

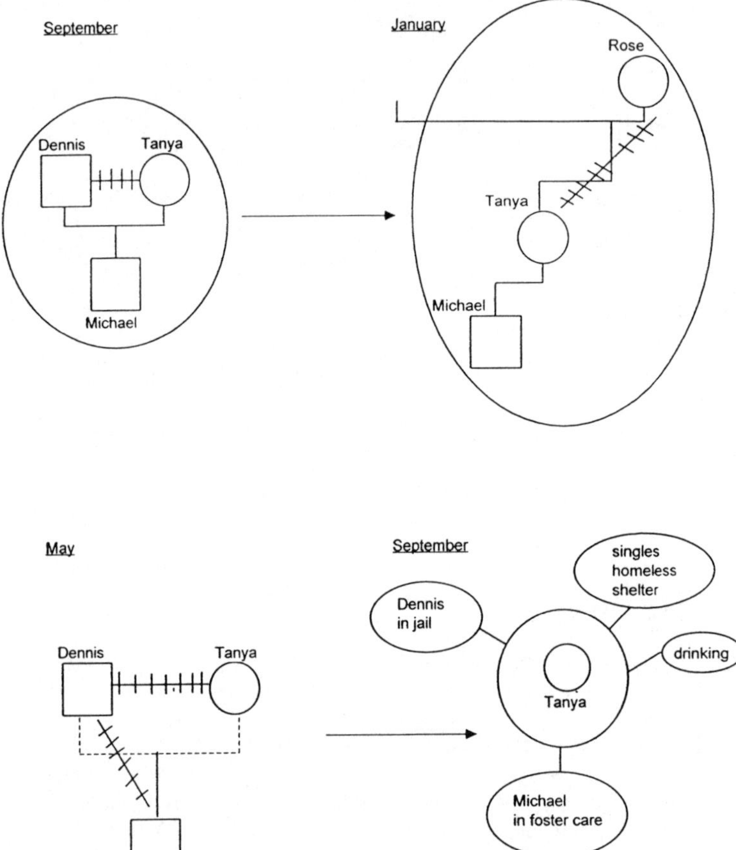

Figure 9.2. Jones Family: Scenario 1 Ecomap

again. Dennis also began to direct his frustration and anger toward Michael, on several occasions slapping and spanking him for "crying too much." Tanya considered returning to her grandmother's home but hesitated, as Rose was struggling with chemotherapy treatments for her cancer.

In early September, Tanya returned from work one morning to find Dennis gone and Michael crying in his crib with a bruised eye. She took him to the emergency room of a nearby hospital, where he was held while a worker from the state child protective services agency was called. Tanya refused to cooperate with the worker, wanting to "protect" Dennis. But Dennis had been picked up again for possession of drugs. In addition, Tanya learned that they were being evicted from their apartment for non-payment of rent.

Michael was placed in foster care; Rose refused to let Tanya back in her home because she had "let the family down" by not taking adequate care of Michael. Rose also threatened to try to get custody of Michael herself. Thus, Tanya felt that her only alternative was to move into a singles' homeless shelter, where she began drinking heavily to ease her rage and thoughts of suicide.

Scenario 2

One possible alternative to Scenario 1 is depicted in Figure 9.3. At the time of Michael's birth, Tanya was referred by hospital social work staff to a family service agency in Leroy and Rose's neighborhood, within walking distance of their home. Karen, an agency social worker, visited Tanya in the hospital and was able to meet Dennis, who was visiting his new son. Shortly after Tanya and Michael were discharged "home" to stay with Tanya's grandmother, Rose, Karen arranged to make a home visit. Because Rose had "heard about" the neighborhood-based, community-focused family service agency and had talked to a friend who had attended a meeting the agency had held with neighbors about some new programs being developed—including a new health clinic and a home ownership program, Rose, albeit reluctantly, agreed to meet with Karen and Tanya.

After two visits with Tanya and Rose, Karen was able to meet with Tanya and Dennis at the agency and then arranged another home visit that was attended, at Karen's request, by Leroy, Rose, Tanya, and Dennis. At this meeting, Karen talked with each family member about their hopes for themselves and for Michael. Because of previous work by the agency in developing neighborhood-based resources, and based on interests expressed by each family member, Karen was able to get both Dennis and Tanya into a new computer skills training course located in a rehabbed building about half a mile from Rose and Leroy's home. Fees for the course were paid with funding through the state's AFDC JOBS program. Dennis also enrolled in an evening General Equivalency Diploma (GED) course at the local elementary school. When she felt well enough, Rose provided child care for Michael; Michael could also be cared for in the neighborhood day care center sponsored by Rose's church, where his fees were subsidized through JOBS program funding.

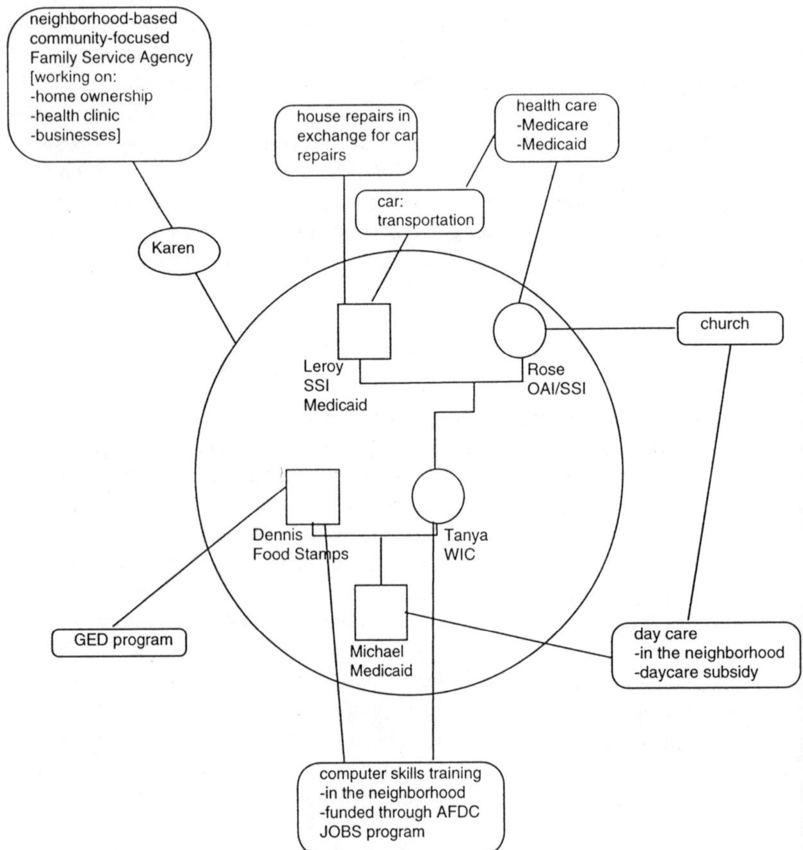

Figure 9.3. Jones Family: Scenario 2 Ecomap

Karen also facilitated Tanya's application for a WIC subsidy. As Karen continued to work with the family, Leroy moved back into the home permanently, and he and Rose invited Dennis to move in with them, provided he and Tanya married, which they subsequently did. Dennis also applied for and received food stamps for his family.

Leroy began working with a group in the community providing transportation for neighborhood residents. He drove Rose to health care appointments and to the social security office to apply for her social security and Medicare benefits. On days when it was raining or very cold, he often drove Dennis and Tanya to their training program. In return for transportation and car repairs for other neighbors, he was able to locate—through the family service agency's "resource and time-exchange bank"—a neighbor who was willing to do some house repairs on a "barter" basis.

Until Dennis and Tanya find jobs that enable them to move out on their own on a stable basis, Leroy and Rose, with occasional supportive discussions with Karen, are willing to have them and Michael continue to live with them. Although this sometimes results in disagreements about how "best to raise" Michael, so far the three-generation household is working out reasonably well.

Tanya's hope is that she and Dennis will soon be able to participate in the agency's home ownership program, through sweat equity in rehabilitating one of the neighborhood houses. The family service agency is also working on attracting businesses into or near the neighborhood, so that parents can walk or take public transportation to work. Michael currently is growing and thriving in a stable pattern of parental and great-grandparental care, along with quality neighborhood day care.

It is clear that poverty in families is a national—as well as a global—social problem which requires macrolevel developmental strategies for change. Such strategies must include policies at state, national, and even international social systems levels. At the same time, family-focused direct service practitioners have vital roles to play in documenting more precisely the extent, the causes, and the consequences of poverty, as well as participating in the development and evaluation of programs to effectively address poverty and related problems in work with low-income families (Janzen & Harris, 1986). Here, I begin with discussion of tools for family assessment and interventions, including identification of several arenas that are critical in further knowledge building. Next, I delineate strategies for social change, including a brief overview of some emerging policy agendas. The chapter concludes with discussion of direct service practitioners' involvement in neighborhood and community knowledge building and development of community- and neighborhood-based interventions for positive social change.

TOOLS FOR FAMILY ASSESSMENT AND INTERVENTIONS

As discussed in Chapter 8, emerging empirically based theory suggests that increasing attention must focus on *both* structural social systems *and* individual and family factors—for example, using Rank's

(1994) structural vulnerability explanation of poverty—to understand and work with families experiencing the stress and potentially catastrophic stress pileup of poverty. As poverty rates increase in the U.S. national social system, it is highly unrealistic for either family members such as the Joneses or social work practitioners such as Karen (in, e.g., child protective services, welfare agencies, mental health clinics, family service agencies, or neighborhood-based or other organizations serving populations in poverty) to expect that change exclusively at the *family* social system level will "solve" the problems faced by families stressed by poverty. On the other hand, to expect major positive changes in larger systems to be developed overnight is also unrealistic. What appears to be necessary is the development of an increasing body of empirically based knowledge from which to develop policies and programs for lasting positive change at multiple social systems levels. To begin, I focus in this section on areas for microlevel knowledge building with and on behalf of families stressed by poverty, using individual and family system tools for both assessment and evaluation of interventions.

Knowledge Building in Direct Practice

The major tools for family assessment—discussed in Chapters 3, 5, and 7—are focused on family system functioning and have been developed to facilitate family-level change. In addition, they can be used by practitioners like Karen, in collaboration with families and with other professionals, (a) to facilitate increased knowledge building regarding ways in which families in poverty do and do not differ from higher-income families; and (b) to track positive or negative change at the family level related to program and policy interventions at larger systems levels (e.g., changes in national health care policy, welfare reform at national and state levels, implementation of school- and neighborhood-based family services). Especially with families stressed by poverty such as Tanya and Dennis, practice must—where possible—be focused *both* (a) on helping families build on their strengths as they struggle with daily survival issues, *and* (b), if families are willing to share their experiences (or to allow their experiences to be shared through appropriate use of group data), on developing empirically based theory and interventions aimed toward systematic knowledge building for effective practice.

Based on the multilevel social systems and stress and coping framework, family-focused practitioners like Karen, in collaboration with other family service agency staff and perhaps also with researchers at a nearby university, can play key roles in further knowledge building in a number of critical areas:

1. Explorations are needed of both the *extent* and the *dynamics* of poverty in families. For example, how do families respond to severe poverty (extremely low income levels)? Is severe poverty (little or no income) different from poverty near the poverty line (income around 95%-99% of the poverty line)? How realistic is the federal poverty line for measuring a frugal, decent standard of living? What difference, if any, does intermittent (in-and-out of) poverty versus "stable" poverty make?
2. How do families "survive" in poverty? For example, what *resources* do they draw upon? What management and social skills are critical for coordinating resources, including employment (often in the secondary labor market), cash benefits, services, family supports, and so forth? Are there particular events that are critical in understanding the destabilization of a family—for example, separation, divorce, family members living in different households because of poverty, involvement with the child welfare system for child neglect or abuse and subsequent placement of a child? Are there critical resources that can make a difference at specific social systems levels—for example, a neighborhood food pantry, periodic or ongoing utility or rent assistance, respite and backup child care from family or friends, stable employment for at least one family member, and so on?
3. What difference, if any, does *time* in poverty make—that is, what are the differences, if any, between families who have had a stable nonpoverty family life and only recently (in the past month or so) experienced below-poverty income levels, versus families who have experienced 3 or more years of chronic (or even intermittent) poverty or are formed by individuals who grew up in poverty?
4. What role do personal and family *beliefs*—as well as health and mental health—play in differentiating families who are more successful in utilizing services and competing for scarce employed-work slots (Rank's, 1994, "chairs")? In social systems in which new resources are actually being created (e.g., job training, jobs, affordable housing, child care services), what types of processes facilitate effective presentation to—and subsequent utilization of—these resources by families and family members?

Tools for Family Assessment

To find—over time—answers to some of the questions posed above, data from a number of the family assessment tools discussed previously can be utilized by Karen and her coworkers at the family service agency.

In particular, use of the following will be discussed briefly: (a) family and household economics; (b) the family ecomap; (c) individual and family time lines; (d) family beliefs, rules, and roles; and (e) measures of individual family members' health and mental health and of family system functioning.

Family and Household Economics. Although a thorough assessment of this aspect of family life is a critical component in understanding and working with families experiencing poverty, obtaining an accurate picture can be both complex and problematic. As shown in Figure 9.4 (and further discussed in Vosler, 1990), the fragmentation of family support programs in the United States results in multiple potential resources—for example, AFDC, housing assistance, food assistance, utilities assistance, emergency assistance, WIC, child support, and child care services. Whether any given family has access to any particular benefit, however, depends on both funding and state and local implementation of an almost-overwhelming variety of policies and programs.

In addition, especially for families such as Dennis and Tanya with at least one family member in the secondary labor market, in which employment may be part-time or temporary, eligibility for one or more benefits may fluctuate dramatically. Because means-testing requirements differ by program, and some programs' cutoff points and income "reductions" depend on the worker's previous month's wages, both eligibility and benefit level may be very different from one month to the next. In such a potentially chaotic income and resource environment, the identification and management of family resources and expenditures becomes very difficult, both for families such as the Joneses and for practitioners such as Karen, as they try to understand resource and service systems. Much more knowledge is needed regarding how the various programs delineated in the Family Access to Basic Resources (FABR) chart (Figure 9.4) interact to support or destabilize family and household economics.

Because most of the income maintenance and many of the social service programs used by families experiencing poverty in the U.S. national social system are means-tested, there are disincentives to report even fairly small economic transactions, such as through barter or other intrafamily or friendship-based support mechanisms. Concomitantly, there may be a reluctance by families and family members to fully disclose all expenses and supports, because to do so might jeopardize a current fragile income-expenses equilibrium. Thus, valid data may

PART 1 - Monthly expenses for a family of this size and composition

Work expenses
- Transportation: $ ________
- Child care: $ ________
- Taxes: $ ________

Purchases for basic needs
- Decent housing: $ ________
- Utilities: $ ________
- Food: $ ________
- Clothing: $ ________
- Personal care: $ ________
- Recreation: $ ________

Health care
- Medical: $ ________
- Dental: $ ________
- Mental health: $ ________
- Special (e.g., substance abuse): $ ________
- Education: $ ________
- Family and developmental (counseling) services: $ ________
- Procurement of resources/services (e.g., transportation): $ ________

Monthly total: $ ________

PART 2 - Potential monthly family resources

Money income
- Wages (If parents' occupations are known, what are average monthly wages for these types of jobs?): $ ________
- Earned Income Tax Credit (EITC): $ ________
- Child support (if applicable): $ ________
- Income transfers (for those unemployed or not expected to work)
  - Unemployment insurance: $ ________
  - Workmen's compensation: $ ________
  - Social Security: $ ________
  - Supplemental Security Income (SSI): $ ________
  - Aid to Families with Dependent Children (AFDC): $ ________
  - Other (e.g., general relief, emergency assistance): $ ________

Credits, goods, and services (free or sliding scale):
- Housing
  - Section 8: $ ________
  - Other housing assistance (e.g., public housing, shelter, hotel/motel): $ ________
  - Utilities assistance: $ ________
- Food
  - Food stamps: $ ________
  - Women's, Infants', and Children's Supplementary Food Program (WIC): $ ________
  - Food bank, food pantry, and other food assistance: $ ________

Monthly total: $ ________

Clothing: Access to used clothing store? Yes ☐ No ☐

Personal care and recreation:
- Access to free recreational facilities? Yes ☐ No ☐

Health care:
- Private Insurance? Yes ☐ No ☐
- Medicare? Yes ☐ No ☐
- Medicaid? Yes ☐ No ☐
- Health clinic? Yes ☐ No ☐
- Dental clinic? Yes ☐ No ☐
- Mental health services? Yes ☐ No ☐
- Special services (e.g., drug abuse treatment)? Yes ☐ No ☐

Education
- Public education? Yes ☐ No ☐
- Special education? Yes ☐ No ☐
- Tutoring? Yes ☐ No ☐
- General Equivalency Diploma (GED)? Yes ☐ No ☐
- Job training? Yes ☐ No ☐

Family and developmental (counseling) services
- Family services? Yes ☐ No ☐
- Support groups? Yes ☐ No ☐
- Family life education? Yes ☐ No ☐

Procurement
- Transportation? Yes ☐ No ☐

PART 3 - Current resources

A. Access to resources last month

Money income
- Wages (use net pay; then subtract other work expenses from Part 1 above, including child care, transportation, etc.): $ ________
- Earned Income Tax Credit (EITC): $ ________
- Child support: $ ________
- Income transfers: $ ________

Credits, goods, and services
- Housing: $ ________
- Food: $ ________
- Clothing: $ ________
- Personal care and recreation: $ ________
- Health care: $ ________
- Education: $ ________
- Family and developmental services: $ ________
- Procurement: $ ________

Monthly total: $ ________

Figure 9.4. Family Access to Basic Resources (FABR)

SOURCE: Vosler (1990, pp. 436-437). Copyright 1990, National Association of Social Workers, Inc., *Social Work.* Used by permission.

depend on practitioners' ability ethically to ensure confidentiality and subsequently to gain the trust of families struggling to survive on often very inadequate resources.

B. Resource stability

How stable was each resource over the past year (very stable, somewhat stable, somewhat unstable, very unstable)? Discuss for each type of resource.

Wages and Earned Income Tax Credit: Overall access to wages through employment? Types of jobs available? Part-time or full-time? Wage levels? Benefits? How would/do you deal with child care or supervision of youth? Quality of child care? Do you have choices? How would/do you deal with an ill child? How would/do you get to and from work? What education and training are needed for good jobs? What education and training opportunities are available? Have you been laid off or terminated or experienced a plant closing? Number of times unemployed? Length of time unemployed? Do you receive the Earned Income Tax Credit (EITC)?

Child support: How is this received? How was the amount decided? Are checks regular? Are payments up to date? Other problems?

Income transfers: What experiences have you had in receiving benefits? What kinds of attitudes have you encountered? How adequate are benefits relative to your family's expenses? Has a check been cut? Has a check been delayed? Have you been dropped from benefits for reasons you didn't understand?

Housing: Rent or own? Choice? Maintenance a problem? Are utilities adequate? Have you been put on a waiting list or been dropped from Section 8 or other housing assistance? Have you had to move or been evicted because the landlord converted to higher rents, condominiums, etc.? Have you experienced homelessness?

Food: Quality? Variety? Have your Food Stamps or WIC been cut or delayed? If so, do you understand why? Has other food assistance been cut or changed?

Clothing: Variety for different roles?

Personal care and recreation: What kinds of recreation? Individual? Family?

Health care: High quality? Choice? Available in a crisis? Have you been dropped from health care coverage with an employer or from Medicaid? If so, why? Have you or another family member been put on a waiting list, for example, for medical or dental care, for counseling for a mental health problem, or for treatment for alcohol or drug abuse? If so, how long did the person have to wait for services?

Education: High quality? Available for all ages? For special needs? Choice? Have you participated in education or training paid for with loans? If so, how are you managing loan repayments?

Family and developmental services: High quality? Choice? Available in a crisis? Have you or another family member been put on a waiting list, for example, for family counseling? If so, how long did the person have to wait for services?

Procurement: Bus? Car? What's within walking distance? How reliable is transportation (e.g., bus and/or car)? How close are bus lines to home, work, child care, shopping, etc.?

Other comments and reflections:

Figure 9.4. Continued

In addition, in some high-poverty and high-crime neighborhoods (see Figure 8.4 and discussion), some families' economic survival may depend at least temporarily on a family member's participation in alternative "underground economies," particularly drug dealing. Practitioners and agencies need to begin to devise understandings and protocols concerning whether to elicit information regarding such activities and resources, and, if so, what ethical guidelines must be followed regarding confidentiality versus neighborhood crime and safety issues and justice system involvement.

The Family Ecomap. As discussed in Chapters 3, 5, and 7 (see also Figure 4.2), the family ecomap is a tool for examining family resources and stressors from—and to—larger systems and structures. Based on the discussion in the previous section, the practitioner and family members might begin to map all of the resource programs with which the family is, or has been, connected, along with positive and negative interactions. An ecomap may reveal that a family is doing an astonishingly good job of managing an array of benefits and resources—each of which individually is a small contribution to the family's economic base but, taken together (and assuming that all are reasonably stable over time) enable the family to survive (Figure 9.5). Alternatively, an ecomap may reveal that a different family (Figure 9.6) is unconnected to potential resources, whether because the resources are unavailable or inaccessible in the neighborhood or community or because family members are disconnected from available resources for a variety of possible reasons (e.g., discriminatory practices built into one or more programs, misunderstandings or difficulties between a family member and a particular program staff member, a family member's depression or other mental health or physical difficulties).

In addition, discussion of an ecomap may reveal that a particular family household is vitally connected economically—possibly in complex ways—to one or more extended-family (or fictive-kin) households as a way of coping with chronic resource deficits. It is possible to theorize that for a few extended-family networks, a kind of "hunting and gathering" survival-focused strategy might develop. This could include (a) one household with some employed-work income in the secondary labor market, (b) an emotionally and financially linked household tapping into as many public assistance resources as possible, and (c) one or more extended-family individuals—especially young and single males or females—engaging in such underground-economy activities as drug dealing or prostitution. Although such a network might be expected to experience instability and potential disaster—a family member seriously diseased (e.g., with AIDS), injured, disabled, ad-

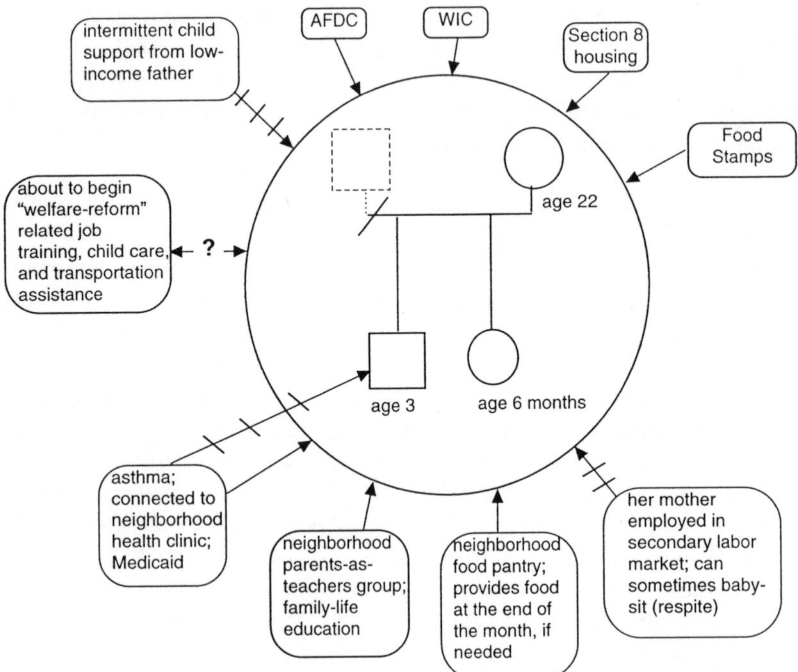

Figure 9.5. Household Ecomap: Family Connected to Resources and Currently Stable

dicted to drugs, jailed, or killed—with increasing stress from chronic poverty, such an interhousehold economy might be experienced by members of the extended-family network as the best-possible solution to the struggle for survival.

Time Lines. Construction and discussion of individual and family time lines and time and tasks management (see Chapters 3, 5, and 7; Figures 3.6, 5.4, and 7.2) can reveal patterns of education; employment and unemployment; and short-term, intermittent, or long-term poverty or near poverty. Families only recently stressed by poverty may find helpful (a) a process of remembering past successes in training programs or job search, and (b) observation of role shifts in the families of

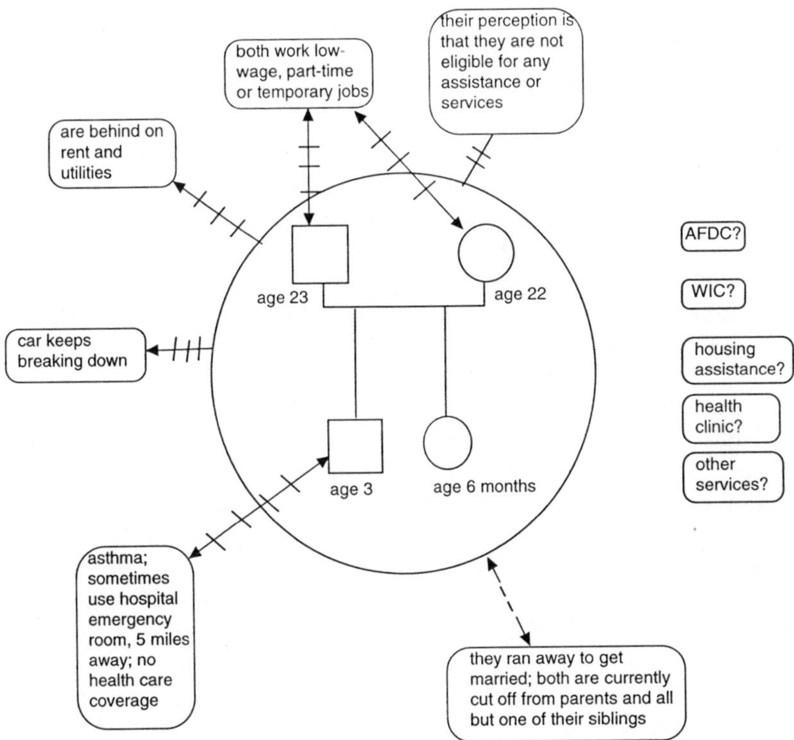

Figure 9.6. Household Ecomap: Family Unconnected to Resources and Stressed

acquaintances or friends who have established new patterns of employed work, family work, and supported child care, whether in an extended-family system or through community services. As indicated in Chapter 8, however, for many families, further education or training programs may have been tried—with a negative outcome of either no job or a job with inadequate wages. Especially if a family member grew up in poverty, education may have been intermittent or terminated early because of survival needs of the family—for example, staying home with siblings or an ill family member, running errands, or part-time work. Seeing a family member's health destroyed by employment in a dangerous secondary labor market job may have influenced a client to distrust employers, leave employment, or not pursue particular employment "opportunities."

Beginning to "walk in the shoes" of family members—particularly when combined with a home visit, a neighborhood walk, and so forth—can alert practitioners like Karen to both the differences and the similarities of living in chronic poverty compared to stable working- or middle-class life. Listening to family members stressed by poverty and helping clients see their own experiences in the context of economic and funding changes in larger social systems can initiate a process of mutual learning and knowledge building between individuals as well as (when information is shared) at larger-system levels.

Family Beliefs. Inevitably, a discussion of family time lines and time and tasks management will illuminate family beliefs, rules, and role expectations. As noted in Chapter 8, as well as in Chapter 4 (see Figure 4.3), the experience of inability to provide successfully for the family's basic needs may result in blaming among family members as well as low self-esteem, frustration and anger, helplessness and hopelessness, depression, and escalating family conflict. Much more data, leading to more valid and comprehensive theoretical understandings, are needed about how family members in a family system chronically stressed by poverty come to view both how the world operates and their ability to control—and therefore take responsibility for—their own lives as well as to influence the functioning of larger systems.

Theoretically, one could posit that in at least some chronically stressed families, there may be a tendency to stabilize in a semidepressed and hopeless worldview—which might be difficult to change until larger-system changes demonstrate the stable availability of resources and opportunities over a fairly long period of time. Thus, even when resources are offered—perhaps depending on how long the old (and previously reinforced) worldview had been in place—it could take a number of years for "multiproblem" (i.e., multistressed) families to exhibit noticeably stable positive change.

Measures of Health, Mental Health, and Family System Functioning. As noted previously, to identify and track positive, negative, and no-change outcomes for families and family members, related to economic and other changes and to consciously implemented policy and program interventions in larger social systems, valid and reliable measures of individual health (physical as well as mental) and of family system functioning are needed. Researchers and other practitioners using currently available measurement tools must continually evaluate the validity of the measures for the specific populations with which each measurement tool is being utilized. For example, are there differences in how chronically stressed, very low income family members experience or report depressive symptoms as compared to working-class or middle-income individuals (Rocha, 1994)? Are there differences between very low income families and other families in how family conflict is experienced or reported (Rocha, 1994)? Similarly, are there differences—by race, ethnicity, gender, and so on—that affect the validity of findings using current measures? In addition, is it possible to develop tools that can be applied to all kinds of individuals and families? If so, how will they be constructed and who will do this work? If not, what methods for comparing across differences can be developed?

Short- and Long-Term Intervention Planning

As the above discussion implies, work with families experiencing the stress of poverty can be extremely challenging and very frustrating. Short-term interventions to address immediate survival needs are often a necessary first step. But without adequate and stable resources and opportunities for "stable-enough" employment that provides sufficient income for a frugal, decent standard of living, combined with family work community supports (Figure 4.3), practitioners who work with family members in family systems experiencing secondary labor market employment and poverty are likely to find themselves continually frustrated by an ongoing series of crises and negative outcomes.

In addition to meeting short-term needs and building on very real survival strengths of families and their members, practitioners like Karen and family members such as the Joneses must begin to see and understand larger-system realities. Subsequently, they can perhaps begin planfully to share data regarding consequences and costs of current larger-system functioning and structures. They might also collaboratively discuss and plan for multilevel long-term interventions to address the needs of all families for stable access to basic resources. It is clear that such participatory family research, involving strategies and programs designed to effectively address poverty and its related stressors, is itself very challenging, since what to evaluate, in what time frames, by what criteria, and at what level(s) (individual, family, program, agency, neighborhood, etc.) have not yet been established.

STRATEGIES FOR SOCIAL CHANGE

Although most family-focused practitioners have traditionally left social change strategy building to more macro-focused professionals, it is clear that with structural economic changes and increasing poverty in the U.S. national social system, effective micropractice with many individuals and families depends on equally effective strategies for positive social change at state, national, and even international systems levels. Here, I briefly discuss a number of avenues for participation in the creation of strategies for positive social change: (a) accurately perceiving poverty, its causes, and consequences; (b) "common well-being education" efforts; (c) collaborative development of interdisciplinary models for social policy change; (d) advocacy and coalition building; and (e) professional knowledge development.

Perceiving Poverty, Its Causes, and Consequences

As indicated in Chapter 8, there are a number of different ways of viewing poverty, including various explanations of its causes, and therefore of addressing associated problems. As Rank (1994) points out, large numbers of the general public in the United States hold firmly to individualistically oriented beliefs about poverty. These include explanations focusing on "deviant" attitudes, behaviors, and motivations, without taking into account the possibility that such factors, where they exist, might be adaptive responses to structural forces beyond the individual's or family's control. Leaders in social work education and continuing education must insist on empirically based theory and professional knowledge building—such as Rank's (1994) structural vulnerability explanation of poverty—to assist practitioners in both micro- and macropractice to understand current realities and emerging trends.

Too often, the frustration from work with low-income individuals and families can lead microtrained practitioners to "blame the victim" for such realities as multiple crises and survival oriented beliefs that can be found among some multiply-stressed families in chronic poverty. It may be difficult for some practitioners who grew up in middle- or upper-class—or even working-class—families to imagine what it might be like to experience a chronic inability to provide adequately for one's family, pay the rent as well as the utilities, or manage the plethora of program resources that sometimes flow (and sometimes do *not* flow) from social service programs.

Personal and professional commitments are needed with a focus on seeing and understanding both the structural social systems factors and the individual and family factors that are involved as both causes and consequences as increasing numbers of families in the United States are caught in stress from chronic poverty. As Rank (1994) so clearly states, social workers must begin to see and analyze not only the "players" in the "game of musical chairs" that is the current economy and labor market, but also the "game" itself.

"Common Well-Being Education"

As discussed briefly in Chapter 7, social workers must develop ways to participate in "common well-being education"—that is, in education of the voting public ensuring understanding of multiple levels of social systems, poverty, and the impacts (in stress pileup and destabilization) of financial strain and deprivation on individuals and families (Voydanoff, 1991) as well as on neighborhoods and local communities. Given the individualistic orientation of belief systems in the United States, ways of helping concerned citizens grasp current and emerging realities need to be developed, such as Rank's (1994) musical chairs and Monopoly game analogies (i.e., persons born into upper-income families begin the current capitalistic Monopoly game of life with "$5,000," middle-income players with "$1,500," and low-income players with "$250," with fairly predictable long-term odds for outcomes—see p. 181). In addition, working with journalists and other media personnel, professionals can help to disseminate and discuss (a) information on the long-term costs of maintaining—or of changing in negative directions—structures in the current economic "game"; (b) findings regarding successful interventions and programs; and (c) promising new policy and program proposals that are based on empirically based theories and models, and on an understanding that there is enough for a frugal, decent standard of living for all citizens in the United States.

Interdisciplinary Model Development

In addition to participation in personal and public education efforts, practitioners can become involved in the collaborative development of interdisciplinary models for social policy change. A number of family and poverty policy proposals have been—and continue to be—discussed in a variety of social science and policy literatures (see, e.g., Chelf, 1992; Chilman, 1988b; Edelman, 1987; Ellwood, 1988; Garfinkel, 1992; Hartman, 1993; Ozawa, 1991; Rank, 1994; Rodgers, 1990; Schorr, 1988; Shapiro & Greenstein, 1993; Sherraden, 1991; etc.). As various aspects of these proposals are enacted and implemented, family-focused practitioners have a vital role to play in documenting both positive and negative outcomes—and intended and unintended consequences—of policy changes. In this section, I summarize policy models proposed by Ellwood (1988) and by Rank (1994). A brief discussion of some additional components of proposals from several other authors follows.

Ellwood's (1988) Policy Model. Because at least some elements of David Ellwood's (1988) policy model are currently influencing the development of a U.S. national policy agenda—particularly with regard to welfare reform and poverty—I discuss the model in some detail. Ellwood begins by identifying four fundamental U.S. "value tenets" (i.e., national beliefs) that "seem to underlie much of the philosophical and political rhetoric about poverty": (a) the "autonomy of the individual," (b) the "virtue of work," (c) the "primacy of the family," and (d) the "desire for and sense of community" (p. 16). Based on these values and following a thorough analysis of poverty for each of three different kinds of families (i.e., two-parent families, single-parent families, and families experiencing urban "ghetto poverty"), Ellwood makes a series of policy proposals.

First, he states, "I believe that in a two-parent family, the earnings of one person working full year, full time (or the equivalent number of hours of combined work by a husband and wife) ought to be sufficient for a family to reach the poverty line" (Ellwood, 1988, p. 87). This proposal implicitly recognizes the importance of time and energy for family work and does not rely on the assumption of a traditional, gender-based division of provider versus family manager.

To implement this policy direction for families—with particular attention to current low-income working-poor families—Ellwood (1988) proposes four specific policy components: (a) "ensure that everyone has medical protection," (b) "make work pay," (c) "replace welfare and food stamps with transitional assistance of a limited duration," and (d) "provide a limited number of jobs for those who have exhausted their transitional assistance" (p. 105). As part of "making work pay," he proposes (a) policies to ensure economic "growth and productivity" (p. 109)—including programs that stimulate economic growth, provide relevant training and education for workers, and ensure access to work experience; (b) raising the minimum wage or experimenting with wage subsidies; (c) expansion of the Earned Income Tax Credit (EITC); and (d) "other steps" (p. 116)—such as a refundable child care credit, a children's allowance, or a children's refundable tax credit.

Developing his discussion of working-poor two-parent families, Ellwood (1988) notes, "It is not one factor, but all three in interaction—labor market difficulties, the dual role [i.e., employed work and family work] of single mothers, and the nature of the welfare system—that create the often impossible situation of many single mothers" (p. 150). He therefore proposes, "The goal should be to *replace* welfare with something that gives people real options, a real chance to be independent, and a real reason to work" (p. 155). He begins with a focus on "reasonable expectations of absent parents" (p. 156), including (a) "identifying every child's father and mother," (b) expecting all absent parents "to contribute a portion of their income (earnings), . . . [using] a roughly uniform formula"; and (c) "payments . . . collected by employers just like Social Security taxes" (p. 163). He also endorses Garfinkel's proposal for a child support assurance system whereby, "When the collections from the earnings of the absent parent were insufficient to provide some minimum level of child support, . . . the government would provide that minimum" (Garfinkel, cited in Ellwood, 1988, p. 165). Ellwood goes on to state, "If child support assurance was combined with the measures suggested . . . [previously]—medical protection, a higher minimum wage, an expanded earned income tax credit (EITC), and a refundable child care credit—the options available to single mothers would be changed dramatically" (p. 166). For single-parent families, he argues, "No one who is willing to work half time . . . [should] have an income below the poverty line" (p. 180). It should be noted, however, that he does not discuss the possible difference between poverty-line income and *stable,* adequate employment and income providing at least a *frugal, decent standard of living* as a foundation that is necessary for family members to create and maintain stable, healthy families (Voydanoff, 1991).

Finally, in discussing the devastation of "ghetto poverty," Ellwood (1988) proposes, in addition to the policies delineated above, "a multifaceted approach" (p. 220) that might include education and training, direct creation of jobs, "empowerment" (p. 223), "teach[ing] responsibility and values" (p. 224), "impos[ing] obligations" (p. 226), and addressing "desegregation and integration" dilemmas (p. 228). In summary,

> A set of social policies that ensure that all families who are willing to work a reasonable level will be secure, autonomous, and responsible for their own decisions seems essential if we are to begin the process of healing the desperation in America's inner cities.
>
> We must not stop there. Education, empowerment, jobs, the teaching of values and responsibility, and one-to-one services all must be a part of a larger strategy to give people a genuine sense of options for the future, a sense of control, and a feeling of being part of, not isolated from, the larger society. (pp. 229-230)

Rank's (1994) Policy Model. In a somewhat parallel set of proposals, Rank (1994) recommends the following social policies to address welfare reform and the national problem of poverty:

1. Employment policies "to produce low levels of unemployment, creating jobs with livable wages and benefits, and to prepare people to fill such jobs" (p. 188)
2. Asset-development policies recommended by Sherraden (1991) and described briefly in the next section
3. "Tax benefits to assist low-income workers," including, for example, the EITC, refundable child care tax credits, or "a per capita refundable credit" (p. 191)
4. "Policies to buffer the economic consequences of family change" (p. 192), such as child support, education and access to contraception, "motivation" and education, career and income opportunities, and accessible and affordable child care
5. Universal health care
6. "Community resources and opportunities," including policies and programs that strengthen "the major institutions found within lower-income communities," that is, "schools, businesses and industries, lending establishments, community centers, and so on" (p. 194)

In summary, Rank (1994) writes,

> The six approaches just described have the potential to temper and reduce the likelihood of poverty and the need for public assistance. As such, they

> are useful and productive. They include establishing a coordinated employment policy, building individual assets, providing tax benefits to assist low-income workers, addressing the economic consequences of family change, providing universal health care, and developing and building community resources and opportunities. All focus on reducing the number of losers that the overall game produces. . . . However, it must also be emphasized that . . . as long as the current economic, social, and political systems exist in this country, some people will be economically vulnerable. While there are a number of positive aspects about our free market capitalist system, there is also a price—a price that has been exacted in the lives of . . . people. . . . The point is to begin to temper and reduce this price. (pp. 196-197)

Other Policy Components. Additional components of family-focused policy needing further discussion, implementation, and evaluation include (a) Sherraden's (1991) Individual Development Accounts; (b) adequate maternity, paternity, and family leave policies; (c) funding for family life education and personal social services; and (d) redistributive tax policies.

Sherraden (1991) argues persuasively for a shift in focus in addressing poverty and welfare from residual, means-tested policies to a "universal asset-based welfare policy" (p. 221) using "Individual Development Accounts" (IDAs) to enable all citizens—and particularly the poor—to accumulate assets for home ownership, education, retirement, starting a business, and so forth. In addition, he states,

> The ideal role of the federal government in social policy-making is long-term. Policy-making at the national level is not suited to short-term adjustments. . . . Therefore, the primary role of the federal government should be to establish a coherent set of long-term rules and incentives—taxes, expenditures, regulations, and general goals—that will be in the best interest of society as a whole, through all of its ups and downs. . . . Promotion of asset accumulation should be a major part of this long-term social policy strategy. (p. 288)

A number of authors have discussed the need for adequate maternity, paternity, and family leave policies (Chilman, 1988b; Hartman, 1993; Moen, 1992) and have demonstrated their importance and effectiveness in other countries (Kamerman, 1986; Moen, 1989; Rodgers, 1990).

Chilman (1988b) argues that although personal social and psychological services for poor families may appear to be "a useless luxury"

(p. 226), because of poor families' vulnerability to stress pileup from an array of difficulties, "Ideally, public programs should meet the basic survival needs of families and individuals as a primary service and then seek to meet their social/psychological needs as a secondary, but still important, service" (p. 227). Such services should include family life education as well as clinical services for both individuals and families.

Finally, Hartman (1993), in a discussion of "challenges for family policy" in the United States, argues, "There must be major income and resource redistribution through tax and economic reform that will shrink the enormous gap between the rich and the poor" (p. 500). She concludes, "The challenge of creating a just and caring society is enormous, but if our nation is to survive on into the 21st century, there is no other option" (p. 500).

Advocacy and Coalition Building

It is obvious that many of the policy and program agendas delineated above have been previously proposed and discussed in the United States, often without political or legislative success. Part of the problem in the past might be that voting citizens, as well as microfocused professionals, have not necessarily made the connection between macrolevel policy discussions and their day-to-day lives and work (McInnis-Dittrich, 1994). With structural economic changes at the international level that are resulting in (a) losses of primary labor market jobs—particularly in manufacturing—in the United States, and (b) the creation of low-wage part-time or temporary jobs in the secondary labor market, increasing numbers of families—including social workers and other human service professionals—are experiencing stress from larger social-system changes. They may therefore be more open to the need for policies and programs that support and enable stable family life.

Over the past decades, traditional advocacy organizations, such as welfare rights organizations and other grassroots social welfare groups, have demanded rights and waged numerous legislative battles at state and national levels to address the needs of various constituencies. In recent years, NASW has become involved particularly in advocacy and coalition building efforts around health care and welfare reform initiatives.

Too often these efforts have been regarded by many family-focused social workers as unrelated—or at best marginally related—to the daily practice of seeing and working with individuals and families. In the midst of social changes, social workers at all systems levels are needed who see connections among social systems and participate in a variety of ways in case and class advocacy as well as in coalitions designed for developing, enacting, implementing, evaluating, and then modifying, as needed, state and national policies aimed toward achieving positive social change for families and for all citizens.

Professional Knowledge Building

A key to effecting positive social change is the ongoing building of an empirical and comprehensive professional knowledge base to guide both the development and the evaluation of change efforts at multiple systems levels. With particular attention to families, research and continuing theory building are needed in a number of key areas. These include:

1. Studies of the mechanisms by which economic strain and deprivation and employment instability and uncertainty destabilize families
2. Comprehensive studies of short- and long-term economic and social costs of *not* supporting and enabling stable, healthy family life—for example, in increased child welfare costs, youth crime and violence, drug and alcohol abuse, family violence, physical and mental health difficulties, and family breakdown
3. Research identifying what kinds of programs—with what specific components, with which family member(s), at which systems levels (neighborhood, local community, state, nation)—are effective, individually or in combinations, in stabilizing and supporting newly formed families as well as already chronically stressed families and ensuring healthy functioning for all family members and for the family as a social system.

For all of these studies, the variable of time needs to be addressed as well. How long can families survive in chronic poverty before they suffer irreversible breakdown? How long does it take for families of various types to stabilize as they are initially formed—and to restabilize after a breakdown? (See, e.g., Nair, Blake, & Vosler, in press.)

There is much challenging work to be done both in better understanding connections among social systems of various sizes and disseminating evolving knowledge to professionals and citizens. As this process continues to develop, emerging knowledge can be used to create innovative and effective programs and policies at multiple systems levels.

MULTILEVEL INTERVENTIONS AND EVALUATION

It seems likely that for many family-focused practitioners such as Karen, participation in knowledge building and in development and social change efforts in macrosystems may be focused—at least initially—at the neighborhood and local community levels. It is at these systems levels that most practitioners and clients work and live. In addition, the local level is often the key to putting all the pieces together for assessment and evaluation as well as realistic, stable change. In this section, I briefly review (a) some potential roles for family practitioners, and (b) some areas needing both knowledge building and innovative development efforts by groups including not only professionals but also clients and citizens as collaborative partners.

Practitioner Roles

As indicated in Chapter 7, family practitioners like Karen can play a variety of roles in knowledge building and change efforts—both as professionals and as citizens—in agencies as well as in neighborhoods and local community organizations. In efforts to deal with families such as Dennis and Tanya, stressed by poverty-level income, social workers might begin to channel at least some of their time and energy (and frustration?) into locating, developing, and participating in emerging school-based or community-based family-support programs in low-income neighborhoods in which clients live (see, e.g., Lightburn & Kemp, 1994). Such programming is designed to provide "comprehensive services to families" (p. 16). To be stable and effective, such programs need to be developed and evaluated in collaboration with clients as consumers—and with neighborhood citizens.

Depending on practitioners' interests and skills, roles in larger systems—in agencies and perhaps with university collaboration—could focus more on knowledge building through (a) developing and testing relevant family- and community-level measures for needs assessment and documentation of changes (both positive and negative); (b) designing and implementing a variety of studies, to analyze existing data and to systematically collect and analyze additional data, for understanding processes, program impacts, and individual and family outcomes in a variety of neighborhoods and communities; and (c) actively participating in larger studies to compare and contrast program and policy impacts in various types of neighborhood and community contexts.

In addition, practitioners—including researchers, administrators, and educators—are needed to develop collaborative avenues for effectively disseminating program and research findings (a) among the general public, (b) at professional social work and interdisciplinary conferences and gatherings, and (c) in the education and training of social work students—who are the next generation of practitioners.

Stable, Comprehensive Local and Neighborhood Development

It is clear that there is a need for an increasing focus on the development of stable, healthy neighborhoods and local communities. Family practitioners like Karen in neighborhood-based family service agencies have vital roles to play in both development efforts and in knowledge building about a variety of local social systems. As Coulton and Pandey (1992) point out in their study of census tract data from the city of Cleveland and surrounding suburbs, there seem to be differences even between low-income neighborhoods: "Geographic areas differed in the incidence of low birth weight, infant death, teen pregnancy, delinquency, and poor reading scores in primary grades. Although high-poverty areas had a higher incidence of these conditions, poor areas were not homogeneous" (p. 254). They conclude, "Not all poor areas display high risk for children, only those with substantial numbers of crimes, female-headed households, or substandard dwellings" (p. 253).

As discussed in Chapters 3 and 5, it is often the microfocused practitioner with data from home visits and a neighborhood walk who can provide critical data for understanding the mechanisms by which families and neighborhoods are caught in maladaptive—versus developing bonadaptive—social processes and structures. For families to function in healthy ways, the surrounding social systems must provide not only accessible and high-quality traditional social services, such as child welfare and juvenile justice services; health, substance abuse, and mental health services; child and family services; elderly services; and public assistance (i.e, income maintenance) benefits. In addition, the entire local community as a social system—including neighborhoods—must be assessed with a focus on employment, wage levels, housing (including utilities) and its quality and affordability, transportation systems, location of neighborhood institutions (schools, banks, clinics, retail shops, repair and maintenance services, businesses, industries, a variety of social services, etc.), voting patterns and political participation, continuing education and training and retraining, affordable quality child care and other dependent care services, and preventive services (e.g., family life education, prevention of crime and violence, and support of a variety of neighborhood associations and organizations).

Thus, neighborhood and local community development—such as the work being facilitated by the family service agency in the Jones family's neighborhood—must include comprehensive social systems analysis that involves looking at *integrated social development.* This will involve not only traditional social services but also economic development and structures for local participation and stable maintenance. In addition, tools and models for effective involvement in integrated social development must be created, tested, evaluated, refined, and disseminated. Such knowledge-building efforts—enabling participation both by professionals with a variety of skills and expertise as well as by neighborhood clients and residents (see Graber, Haywood, & Vosler, in press)—are critical in understanding and effectively addressing complex social problems associated with economic change and increasing poverty in the United States as well as internationally.

SUMMARY

To work effectively with the increasing numbers of families experiencing stress pileup from poverty, social workers and other human service professionals must include in their work not only family- and neighborhood-focused interventions but also participation in strategies for social change at more macro social systems levels. Such strategies can include "common well-being education" for all citizens, advocacy and coalition building, and development of consensus through professional knowledge building. The development of effective interdisciplinary models for multilevel social systems change is an ongoing enterprise. Through social service agencies and through collaboration with universities and other research organizations, practitioners at all levels can and must make a difference in solving the problem of poverty and the accompanying devastation of neighborhoods, families, and family members.

Chapter 10

EPILOGUE AND CONCLUSIONS

EPILOGUE

Andrew Billingsley, a family scholar and author of *Climbing Jacob's Ladder: The Enduring Legacy of African-American Families* (1992) as well as a number of other books focusing on both strengths and constraints in the lives of African Americans, has observed that in-depth understandings of complex social phenomena often require three "methods": statistics, studies, and stories (Billingsley, 1995). In this vein, I offer the following story:

> Once there was a very beautiful land, with mountains, lakes, rivers, and rain in abundance. Early on, diverse groups established a variety of societies, some building homes in the mountains, others growing crops by the rivers, and still others following the buffalo on the plains. The rain fell on all of the groups, and there was enough.
>
> Later, other people moved onto the land, each household claiming "my" small piece of the rivers' or lakes' waterfronts. Changes in the prevailing winds resulted in the rain falling only high up in the mountains, and in time, all of the water for sustaining people's lives came only from the lakes and rivers—not directly from rain.
>
> As a result of this change, some people along the river began to worry about "having enough" to sustain life—especially as more and more people came. Soon, all of the lake- and riverfront properties were claimed. Technology was created for building dams in the mountains and along the rivers to "manage" the flow of resources. It was also discovered that

aqueducts could be built from the rivers to places where people who had no waterfront property could be sustained. The families living at the end of the aqueducts tended to be elderly people, children and their parents, persons with disabilities, and the descendants of former slaves, who had been denied waterfront properties when they had arrived because they were slaves.

With advances in technology, people also began to build beautiful fountains, elaborate swimming pools, and lawns and golf courses that required frequent watering to keep them lush and green. People who lived around the lakefronts were especially blessed with access to an abundance of water.

One day, the people who lived downstream along the rivers, far from the mountains and lakes, began to notice that the water level in the river had dropped. They anxiously monitored the water in the river; and, although there were still the normal up-and-down fluctuations, the long-term trend was toward less and less water flowing into the lower reaches of the rivers.

Concern mounted. There were many families living along the rivers who depended on the rivers for life. Without water to sustain them, lives would be in jeopardy. One day, a spokesperson emerged who announced a startling revelation—that the problem facing the lower-river people was simply that the aqueducts were siphoning off too much water. Therefore, the obvious solution to the problem was that the aqueducts should be torn down, and the "dependent people" at the end of the aqueducts should be told to go find their own water.

The end of this story has not yet been written.

CONCLUSIONS

From the summaries of statistics and studies regarding families, work, unemployment, and poverty reviewed in the previous chapters of this book, I draw several major conclusions for consideration and use by social workers and other human service professionals who work with and on behalf of families particularly in U.S. society today:

1. Families, especially families with children, are under increasing stress and at risk of catastrophic stress pileup from poverty because of loss of high-wage jobs from the national economy and stagnant or falling wages for many—particularly disadvantaged—workers. For many families with children, it takes two full-time wage earners to provide for the family's basic necessities, potentially leading to role overload

for parents—or caregivers of elderly or disabled family members—who must juggle three full-time "jobs": two full-time-equivalent provider roles and one full-time-equivalent family work role. In this larger-system environment, jobs, wages, and high-quality, accessible and affordable community supports are key to enabling families to achieve goals of stable family life and healthy living for all family members, including children.

2. Given changes in economic systems, particularly at national and global levels, the multilevel social systems model discussed in this book is a critical tool for assessment and intervention planning, including policy and program development in work with families, particularly families stressed by the struggle to provide adequately and stably for all family members.

The story at the beginning of this chapter indirectly asserts that there is enough water for all families to have their basic needs met—that is, we as a society in the United States know how to grow food, make clothing, build housing, and train health care workers and teachers to ensure a decent, frugal standard of living for every citizen in every family. But as Rank (1994) notes, we must analyze not only the family who comes to ask for help but also the "game" represented by the current structures of our society—at local, state, and national as well as global levels—to discern who needs to change, in what directions, toward what goals, through what policies and rule changes, with what results. No longer can social workers and other human service professionals assume that helping the family to change will "solve" problems of role overload, unemployment, and poverty. Beyond individual and family assessment, analysis must be broadened to include understandings of how neighborhoods, local communities, and larger systems operate to support or disadvantage families and their members. Based on these multilevel assessments, innovations in social development in larger systems must be made a vital part of the work of social work practice in agencies and organizations—so that work with families can be effective.

3. Theoretical understandings of how social systems operate and change continue to emerge, based on a variety of social science tools and methods (see Chapter 1). As program and policy innovations are designed, studies of their effectiveness, resulting in expanding procedural knowledge, must become a routine part of implementation. As changes are effected, unintended consequences—both positive and

negative—must be discerned, and new propositional knowledge must be developed and disseminated for use by practitioners and citizens alike. Thus, social science knowledge development must become a normal part of social life—an ongoing and continuous enterprise—for social system members at multiple levels from the family to the globe, to see the systems that are continually being constructed and reconstructed and to decide how best to participate in creating structures that enable healthy life for all involved.

4. To do effective work, social workers and other human service professionals must educate not only ourselves but also consumers and other citizens. Just as the public health movement has helped to educate citizens regarding realities and needed changes in individual and community health practices, through "common well-being education" we must communicate the importance of all social system members' understanding economic, political, and cultural realities as well as disseminate knowledge about effective policy, program, and other practice innovations to ensure healthy social development at multiple levels.

It is clear that this vision—of participation in reconstructing social structures and systems to ensure healthy living for all—is not easily accomplished. In fact, it is extremely difficult and frustrating work. But as the story at the beginning of this chapter makes clear, in a global economy, we truly are all in this together. The challenge posed by the multilevel social systems model is to help one another—practitioners and fellow citizens alike—to see both that change is already occurring and that we can and must begin to influence that change in the direction of positive interaction that enables nations, states, local communities, and neighborhoods to support healthy families. Such work benefits not only the social systems in which we work and live but ultimately ourselves, our children, and our children's children as far into the future as we can envision.

APPENDIX

ANG MO KIO
FAMILY SERVICE CENTRES
RESEARCH FORMS

Developed by Nair, Blake, and Vosler (1993). Also being used, with permission, is an adapted form of Taynor, Nelson, and Daugherty's (1990) Family Intervention Scale.

Included are:

- Time 1 (Intake), Form 1
- Time 1 (Intake), Form 2
  - Time 2 (6 Months), Form 1
  - Time 3 (1 Year), Form 1
  - Case Closing, Form 2
- Time 2 (6 Months), Time 2
  - Time 3 (1 Year), Form 2
  - Case Closing, Form 3
- Case Closing, Form 1

Time 1 (Intake), Form 1

ID#: _____________

Family: _____________

Worker: _____________

Date opened (mo/yr): _____________

Reopened?: _____ Yes (1)
_____ No (New case) (0)

Referral source (Please check one only):
_____ Husband (1)
_____ Wife (2)
_____ Child (3)
_____ Other family member (4)
_____ Friend (5)
External System:
_____ HDB (6)
_____ PUB (7)
_____ Town Council (8)
_____ School (9)
_____ Hospital (10)
_____ Police (11)
_____ MP (12)
_____ Other (Please specify: _____________) (13)

Who made the 1st contact? (Please check one only):
_____ The family (1)
_____ AMKFSC (0)

For the initial contact, where was/were family member(s) seen? (Please check one only):
_____ Family's home (0)
_____ AMKFSC (1)
_____ Other (Please specify: _____________) (9)

Presenting problem (Please check one only):
_____ HDB arrears (1)
_____ Financial (2)
_____ Family/marital (3)
_____ Behavioral (4)
_____ Childcare/BASIC (5)
_____ Employment (6)
_____ Other (Please specify: _____________) (7)

Husband's Ethnicity (Please circle one only):

1. Chinese
2. Malay
3. Indian
4. Eurasian
5. Other (Please specify: ______________________________)

Wife's Ethnicity (Please circle one only):

1. Chinese
2. Malay
3. Indian
4. Eurasian
5. Other (Please specify: ______________________________)

Time 1 (Intake), Form 2
Time 2 (6 Months), Form 1
Time 3 (1 Year), Form 1
Time 4 (2 Years), Form 1
Case Closing, Form 2

[Please circle one above]

ID#: ______________

Family Intervention Scale:
- Family Roles
- Social Support
- Physical Maintenance
- Community Resources
- Emotional Well-Being

(Please check if form has been turned in): _____

Date of birth (mo/yr):
- Husband: _____ / _____
- Wife: _____ / _____

Date of Birth:	Gender (circle one):
Child #1 ______ / ______	m / f
Child #2 ______ / ______	m / f
Child #3 ______ / ______	m / f
Child #4 ______ / ______	m / f
Child #5 ______ / ______	m / f
Child #6 ______ / ______	m / f
Child #7 ______ / ______	m / f
Child #8 ______ / ______	m / f
Child #9 ______ / ______	m / f
Child #10 ______ / ______	m / f

Total number of members in current household: _________

(Breakdown of this Total:)

Husband?	______	Yes	(1)
	______	No	(0)
Wife?	______	Yes	(1)
	______	No	(0)

# of their children: ______

# of extended family *adults:* ______

# of extended family *children:* ______

Other (Please specify: ________________): ______

Total monthly household expenses: $ __________
(Breakdown of this Total monthly household expenses:)
Housing/HDB: $ __________
Utilities/PUB: $ __________
SC/CC: $ __________
Telephone: $ __________
Marketing/Food: $ __________
Groceries: $ __________
Transportation:
For work: $ __________
For school: $ __________
For other: $ __________
Childcare: $ __________
Education:
School fees: $ __________
Other school expenses/allowances $ __________
Medical: $ __________
Clothing, personal care: $ __________
Other (e.g., family obligations, debt or loan repayment(s), lunch(es) at work, family outings, recreation):
Please specify:
___________________________ $ __________
___________________________ $ __________
___________________________ $ __________
___________________________ $ __________

Total monthly household cash income: $ __________
(Breakdown of this Total monthly household cash income:)
Husband: $ __________
Wife: $ __________
From other family member(s): $ __________
Subsidy (e.g., P.A.): $ __________
Other:
(Please specify: ____________) $ __________

Monthly household cash income range:
Lowest monthly household cash income: $ __________
Highest monthly household case income: $ __________

Non-financial assistance? (e.g., food, child-care): ______ No (0)
______ Yes (1)

Total household debts: $ __________

Marital status (Please circle one only):

1. Married 2. Widowed
3. Divorced 4. Separated
5. Never married
6. Other (Please specify: ______________________________)

Did either family-of-origin object to the marriage?: ______ No (0)
______ Yes (1)

Husband's religion (Please circle one only):

1. Muslim 2. Hindu
3. Buddhist 4. Taoist
5. Jewish 6. Christian: Catholic
7. Christian: Protestant 8. No religion
9. Other (Please specify: ______________________________)

Wife's religion (Please circle one only):

1. Muslim 2. Hindu
3. Buddhist 4. Taoist
5. Jewish 6. Christian: Catholic
7. Christian: Protestant 8. No religion
9. Other (Please specify: ______________________________)

Husband's education (Please circle one only):

1. No formal education 2. Primary
3. Secondary, 'N' level 4. Secondary, 'O' level
5. 'A' level 6. VITB
7. Polytechnic 8. University
9. Other (Please specify: ______________________________)

Wife's education (Please circle one only):

1. No formal education 2. Primary
3. Secondary, 'N' level 4. Secondary, 'O' level
5. 'A' level 6. VITB
7. Polytechnic 8. University
9. Other (Please specify: ______________________________)

Citizenship:

Husband a Singapore Citizen?: ______ Yes (1)
______ No (0)

Wife a Singapore Citizen?: ______ Yes (1)
______ No (0)

Flat Type (Please circle one only):

1. One room 2. Two room
3. Three room 4. Four room
5. Five room
6. Other (Please specify: ______________________________)

Own or rent? (Please check one only): ______ rent (0)
______ own (1)

Husband's current occupation (Please circle one only):

1. Professional
2. Technical
3. Sales & clerical
4. Craftsman, such as electrician, plumber
5. Production
6. Service, such as police, hospital attendant, beautician
7. Manual, such as cleaner, sweeper, grasscutter
8. Homemaker
9. Retired
10. Student (in school)
11. Other (Please specify: ______________________________)

Wife's current occupation (Please circle one only):

1. Professional
2. Technical
3. Sales & clerical
4. Craftsman, such as electrician, plumber
5. Production
6. Service, such as police, hospital attendant, beautician
7. Manual, such as cleaner, sweeper, grasscutter
8. Homemaker
9. Retired
10. Student (in school)
11. Other (Please specify: ______________________________)

Husband's current employment (Please circle one only):

1. Regular wage earner
2. Unemployed and looking for work
3. Unemployed and not looking for work
4. Part-time wage earner
5. Irregular wage earner
6. Homebased wage earner
7. Other (Please specify: ______________________________)

Wife's current employment (Please circle one only):

1. Regular wage earner
2. Unemployed and looking for work
3. Unemployed and not looking for work
4. Part-time wage earner
5. Irregular wage earner
6. Homebased wage earner
7. Other (Please specify: ______________________________)

General Problems Checklist (Please check ALL that apply):

I. Family, marital, and parental roles:

______ Marital conflict
______ Extra-marital relationship(s)
______ Isolated adolescent parents
______ Communication problems
______ Unplanned children
______ Spousal abuse
______ Physical fighting between parents (violence)
______ School difficulties (child)
______ Child(ren) behavior problem(s)
______ Parent-child conflict
______ Lack of parenting skills (e.g., behavior management, discipline)
______ Physical abuse of child(ren)
______ Sexual abuse of child(ren)

II. Social support:

______ Conflict with extended family member(s)
______ Conflict with workmates
______ Conflict with friends
______ Conflict with neighbors
______ Lack of stable child care
______ Lack of before/after school supervision
______ Conflict with child caregiver(s)
______ Lack of elder care
______ Conflict with elder caregiver(s)
______ Lack of disabled (household member) care
______ Conflict with disabled (household member) caregiver(s)

III. Physical maintenance:

______ Unstable housing (HDB, PUB, Town Council, TELECOM)
______ Debt(s) to family and/or friends
______ Debts and/or credit owed to loan sharks, money lenders, or other creditors
______ Budgeting and/or money management problems
______ Unstable income
______ Household management problem (e.g., unclean apartment, laundry not done)
______ Nutrition problem for child(ren)
______ Nutrition problem for adult(s)
______ Housing maintenance problem (e.g., repairs not done, unsafe environment)

IV. Community resources:

______ Low skills for employment
______ Unemployment
______ Irregular employment
______ Conflict with police or court
______ Conflict with school
______ Conflict with hospital, clinic, or other medical personnel
______ Conflict with employer
______ Conflict with other external systems (e.g., MCD, VWO's);
(Please specify: ______________________________)
______ Transportation problem(s)
(Please specify: ______________________________)
______ Lack of other resources (e.g., banking, legal aid, cultural/recreation opportunities);
(Please specify: ______________________________)

V. Emotional well-being and health:

______ Acute medical problem for adult(s)
______ Chronic medical problem for adult(s)
______ Acute medical problem for child(ren)
______ Chronic medical problem for child(ren)
______ Diagnosed mental illness in adult(s)
______ Diagnosed mental illness in child(ren)
______ Depressed parent(s)
______ Hyperactive child(ren)
______ Learning disabled child(ren)
______ Disabled parent
______ Disabled child(ren)
______ Other disabled family member
______ Alcohol abuse
______ Drug use or addiction
______ Gambling problem
______ Angry outbursts
______ Violent outbursts
______ Expressed sense of hopelessness/helplessness
______ Suicidal ideation/threats
______ Suicide attempt
______ Low IQ (adult)
______ Low IQ (child)
______ Other (Please specify: __________________________)

Systemic Patterns Checklist (household patterns *identified*)
(Please check ALL that apply):

______ Life cycle transition: first child(ren)
______ Life cycle transition: school-aged child(ren)
______ Life cycle transition: adolescent(s)
______ Life cycle transition: launching young adults
______ Life cycle transition: newly married couple
______ Life cycle transition: aging parent(s)' care
______ Entrance(s) into the family
______ Loss (divorce, death)
______ Enmeshed pattern(s)
______ Disengaged/distancing pattern(s)
______ Chaotic/out-of-control pattern(s)
______ Rigid/closed pattern(s)
______ Marital communication unclear
______ Parent-child communication unclear
______ "Mind-reading" statements
______ Parent-child coalition(s)
______ Marital distancing/disengagement
______ Unclear family roles (who does what)
______ Unclear family rules (how things are done)
______ Unrealistic family beliefs
______ Depressed family "mood"
______ Hostile family "mood"
______ Pattern of avoidance
______ Acute unresolved conflict
______ Chronic unresolved conflict
______ Family secrets
______ Other (Please specify: ___________________________)

Time 2 (6 Months), Form 2
Time 3 (1 Year), Form 2
Time 4 (2 Years), Form 2
Case Closing, Form 3

[Please circle one above]

ID#: ______________

Total number of interviews (at least 30 minutes): _____

(Breakdown of this Total—*with whom:*)

All nuclear family members present: _____
Some nuclear members present: _____
Couple only: _____
Nuclear member(s) *plus* extended family and/or friend: _____
Individual: _____
Other (Please specify: ___________________________)

(Breakdown of Total interviews—*where:*)

Home: _____
Office: _____
Other (Please specify: ___________________________)

Social Work Methods Used (Please check ALL that apply):

_____ Client support
_____ Task-oriented (problem-focused) approach
_____ Financial aid (AMKFSC)
_____ Child care (AMKFSC)
_____ BASIC (AMKFSC)
_____ Advocacy and negotiation with external systems
_____ External agencies skills training
_____ Contracting
_____ Referral and follow-up
_____ Household management skills training
_____ Parenting skills training (with 1 person)
_____ Linking
_____ Spousal communication skills training (with 1 person)
_____ Information giving
_____ Other (Please specify: ___________________________)

Systemic Interventions Checklist (Areas worked on/Interventions used)
(Please check ALL that apply):

______ Interpersonal communication training (with 2 or more family members) for clear, direct, empathic/attentive communication
______ Clear consensus on family roles
______ Negotiation, compromise, and conflict resolution training (with 2 or more family members)
______ Clear, "up-to-date" consensus on family beliefs
______ Clear, "up-to-date" consensus on family rules and behaviors
______ Marital cohesion/alliance
______ Appropriate autonomy/connection with families-of-origin
______ Appropriate connecting among family members
______ Repairing cut-offs
______ Separating and letting go
______ Using humor, warmth, and optimism
______ Restructuring family time
______ Redrawing boundaries in physical space
______ Redrawing boundaries in emotional space
______ Reflecting on and supporting change
______ Normalizing
______ Reframing
______ Paradoxical injunctions
______ Other (Please specify: ______________________________)

Client Satisfaction Scale:

1. How satisfied are you with the services or help you have received from the Ang Mo Kio Family Service Centre over the past [6 or 12] months? (Please circle one number only):

Very Satisfied		Moderately Satisfied			Both Satisfied and Dissatisfied		Moderately Dissatisfied		Very Dissatisfied	
11	10	9	8	7	6	5	4	3	2	1

2. How satisfied are you with the work your family and the agency social worker (Name: ________________________) have done over the past [6 / 12] months? (Please circle one number only):

Very Satisfied		Moderately Satisfied			Both Satisfied and Dissatisfied		Moderately Dissatisfied		Very Dissatisfied	
11	10	9	8	7	6	5	4	3	2	1

3. What *suggestions* (if any) do you have to help the agency improve our services to you and other Ang Mo Kio families in the future?:

____

____

____

____

____

____

____

____

____

Case Closing, Form 1

ID#: ______________

Date closed (mo/yr): _____ / _____

At case closing, number of workers assigned
(since case opening): __________

REFERENCES

Aldous, J. (Ed.). (1982). *Two paychecks: Life in dual-earner families.* Beverly Hills, CA: Sage.

Aldous, J., Ganey, R., Trees, S., & Marsh, L. C. (1991). Families and inflation: Who was hurt in the last high-inflation period? *Journal of Marriage and the Family, 53,* 123-134.

Aldous, J., & Tuttle, R. C. (1988). Unemployment and the family. In C. S. Chilman, F. M. Cox, & E. W. Nunnally (Eds.), *Employment and economic problems* (pp. 17-41). Newbury Park, CA: Sage.

Anderson, R. E., & Carter, I. (1990). *Human behavior in the social environment: A social systems approach* (4th ed.). Hawthorne, NY: Aldine de Gruyter.

Angell, R. C. (1936). *The family encounters the Depression.* New York: Scribner.

Armstrong, P. S., & Schulman, M. D. (1990). Financial strain and depression among farm operators: The role of perceived economic hardship and personal control. *Rural Sociology, 55*(4), 475-493.

Babbie, E. (1992). *The practice of social research* (6th ed.). Belmont, CA: Wadsworth.

Bailey, R., & Brake, M. (Eds.). (1975). *Radical social work.* New York: Pantheon.

Bakke, E. W. (1940a). *Citizens without work: A study of the effects of unemployment upon the workers' social relations and practices.* New Haven, CT: Yale University Press.

Bakke, E. W. (1940b). *The unemployed worker: A study of the task of making a living without a job.* New Haven, CT: Yale University Press.

Bank, L., Forgatch, M. S., Patterson, G. R., & Fetrow, R. A. (1993). Parenting practices of single mothers: Mediators of negative contextual factors. *Journal of Marriage and the Family, 55,* 371-384.

Barker, R. L. (1987). *The social work dictionary.* Silver Spring, MD: National Association of Social Workers.

Barnett, R. C., & Baruch, G. K. (1988). Correlates of fathers' participation in family work. In P. Bronstein & C. P. Cowan (Eds.), *Fatherhood today: Men's changing role in the family* (pp. 66-78). New York: John Wiley.

Baum, A., Davidson, L. M., Singer, J. E., & Street, S. W. (1987). Stress as a psychophysiological process. In A. Baum & J. E. Singer (Eds.), *Stress* (Handbook of psychology and health, Vol. 5, pp. 1-24). Hillsdale, NJ: Lawrence Erlbaum.

Baumol, W. J., & Blinder, A. S. (1991). *Microeconomics: Principles and policy* (5th ed.). New York: Harcourt Brace Jovanovich.

Beavers, W. R. (1982). Healthy, midrange, and severely dysfunctional families. In F. Walsh (Ed.), *Normal family processes* (pp. 45-66). New York: Guilford.

Beavers, W. R., & Hampson, R. B. (1990). *Successful families: Assessment and intervention.* New York: Norton.

Beavers, W. R., & Hampson, R. B. (1993). Measuring family competence: The Beavers systems model. In F. Walsh (Ed.), *Normal family processes* (2nd ed., pp. 73-103). New York: Guilford.

Beckett, J. O. (1988). Plant closings: How older workers are affected. *Social Work, 33,* 29-33.

Becvar, D. S., & Becvar, R. J. (1993). *Family therapy: A systemic integration* (2nd ed.). Boston: Allyn & Bacon.

Bellah, R. N., Madsen, R., Sullivan, W. M., Swidler, A., & Tipton, S. M. (1985). *Habits of the heart: Individualism and commitment in American life.* Los Angeles: University of California Press.

Belsky, J. (1990). Parental and nonparental child care and children's socioemotional development: A decade in review. *Journal of Marriage and the Family, 52,* 885-903.

Berardo, F. M. (Ed.). (1980). *Decade review: Family research 1970-1979.* Minneapolis, MN: National Council on Family Relations. [Also published as a special issue of *Journal of Marriage and the Family,* 1980, *42*(4)]

Berry, S., Gottschalk, P., & Wissoker, D. (1988). An error components model of the impact of plant closing on earnings. *Review of Economics and Statistics, 70*(4), 701-707.

Bertalanffy, L. von (1968). *General system theory: Foundations, development, applications.* New York: Braziller.

Biegel, D. E., Cunningham, J., Yamatani, H., & Martz, P. (1989). Self-reliance and blue-collar unemployment in a steel town. *Social Work, 34,* 399-406.

Billingsley, A. (1992). *Climbing Jacob's ladder: The enduring legacy of African-American families.* New York: Simon & Schuster.

Billingsley, A. (1995, January). *African American families: Challenges of uncertainty.* Presentation at the Spring 1995 Lecture Series of the George Warren Brown School of Social Work, Washington University, St. Louis, MO.

Blair, S. L., & Johnson, M. P. (1992). Wives' perceptions of the fairness of the division of household labor: The intersection of housework and ideology. *Journal of Marriage and the Family, 54,* 570-581.

Blair, S. L., & Lichter, D. T. (1991). Measuring the division of household labor. *Journal of Family Issues, 12*(1), 91-113.

Blake, M. (1991). The built environment and the underprivileged. In W. S. J. Lim (Ed.), *Architecture and development in Southeast Asia* [A special issue of *Solidarity* (131-132)], (pp. 87-99). Manila, The Philippines: Solidaridad.

Blake, M. (1993). *1st family session* (Casework forms for Ang Mo Kio Family Service Centres). Singapore: National University of Singapore.

Blake, M., & Lam, S. L. (1993, August). *Family, women and development* (Workshop E). Paper presented at the International Council on Social Welfare Asia-Pacific Regional Conference, Singapore.

Bloom, H. S. (1987). Lessons from the Delaware dislocated worker pilot program. *Evaluation Review, 11*(2), 157-177.

Bloom, M., Wood, K., & Chambon, A. (1991). The six languages of social work. *Social Work, 36*(6), 530-534.

Bluestone, B., & Harrison, B. (1982). *The deindustrialization of America.* New York: Basic Books.

Booth, A. (Ed.). (1991). *Contemporary families: Looking forward, looking back.* Minneapolis, MN: National Council on Family Relations.

Boulding, K. E. (1961). *The image: Knowledge in life and society.* Ann Arbor, MI: University of Michigan Press.

Bowen, M. (1978). *Family therapy in clinical practice.* New York: Jason Aronson.

Bowlby, J. (1969). *Attachment and loss* (Vol. 1, *Attachment*). New York: Basic Books.

Bowlby, J. (1988). *A secure base: Parent-child attachment and healthy human development.* New York: Basic Books.

Boyd-Franklin, N. (1989). *Black families in therapy: A multisystems approach.* New York: Guilford.

Boyd-Franklin, N. (1993). Race, class, and poverty. In F. Walsh, (Ed.), *Normal family processes* (2nd ed., pp. 361-376). New York: Guilford.

Bozett, F. W. (Ed.). (1987). *Gay and lesbian parents.* New York: Praeger.

Brabson, H. V., & Himle, D. P. (1987). The unemployed and the poor: Differing perceptions of their needs in a community. *Social Thought, 13*(1), 24-33.

Brenner, M. H. (1973). *Mental illness and the economy.* Cambridge, MA: Harvard University Press.

Brett, J. M., & Yogev, S. (1988). Restructuring work for family: How dual-earner couples with children manage. In E. Goldsmith (Ed.), *Work and family: Theory, research and applications* (pp. 159-174). Corte Madera, CA: Select Press. [Also published in a special issue of *Journal of Social Behavior and Personality,* 1980, *3*(4), 159-174]

Briar, K. H. (1983). Unemployment: Toward a social work agenda. *Social Work, 28,* 211-216.

Briar, K. H. (1988). *Social work and the unemployed.* Silver Spring, MD: National Association of Social Workers.

Briar, K. H., & Knighton, K. (1988). Helping families with problems of unemployment and underemployment. In C. S. Chilman, F. M. Cox, & E. W. Nunnally (Eds.), *Employment and economic problems* (pp. 43-65). Newbury Park, CA: Sage.

Broderick, C. B. (1993). *Understanding family process: Basics of family systems theory.* Newbury Park, CA: Sage.

Broman, C. L., Hamilton, V. L., & Hoffman, W. S. (1990). Unemployment and its effects on families: Evidence from a plant closing study. *American Journal of Community Psychology, 18*(5), 643-659.

Bronfenbrenner, U. (1979). *The ecology of human development: Experiments by nature and design.* Cambridge, MA: Harvard University Press.

Brown, C. (1983). Unemployment theory and policy, 1946-1980. *Industrial Relations, 22*(2), 164-185.

Brown, D. R., & Gary, L. E. (1985). Predictors of depressive symptoms among unemployed black adults. *Journal of Sociology and Social Welfare, 12,* 736-754.

Brubaker, T. H. (1991). Families in later life: A burgeoning research area. In A. Booth (Ed.), *Contemporary families: Looking forward, looking back* (pp. 226-248). Minneapolis, MN: National Council on Family Relations.

Bumpass, L. L. (1990). What's happening to the family? Interactions between demographic and institutional change. *Demography, 27,* 483-498.

Buss, T. F., & Redburn, F. S. (1983a). *Mass unemployment: Plant closings and community mental health.* Beverly Hills, CA: Sage.

Buss, T. F., & Redburn, F. S. (1983b). *Shutdown at Youngstown: Public policy for mass unemployment.* Albany: State University of New York Press.

Caputo, R. K. (1991). Patterns of work and poverty: Exploratory profiles of working-poor households. *Families in Society, 72*(8), 451-460.

Carter, B., & McGoldrick, M. (Eds.). (1988). *The changing family life cycle: A framework for family therapy.* New York: Gardner.

Cavan, R. S., & Ranck, K. H. (1938). *The family and the Depression: A study of one hundred Chicago families.* Chicago: University of Chicago Press.

Chadiha, L. A. (1992). Black husbands' economic problems and resiliency during the transition to marriage. *Families in Society, 73,* 542-552.

Chelf, C. P. (1992). *Controversial issues in social welfare policy* (Controversial Issues in Public Policy, Vol. 3). Newbury Park, CA: Sage.

Cheung, K. F. M. (1990). Interdisciplinary relationships between social work and other disciplines: A citation study. *Social Work Research & Abstracts, 26*(3), 23-29.

Chilman, C. S. (1988a). Public policies and families. In C. S. Chilman, F. M. Cox, & E. W. Nunnally (Eds.), *Employment and economic problems* (pp. 173-181). Newbury Park, CA: Sage.

Chilman, C. S. (1988b). Public policies and families in financial trouble. In C. S. Chilman, F. M. Cox, & E. W. Nunnally (Eds.), *Employment and economic problems* (pp. 183-236). Newbury Park, CA: Sage.

Chilman, C. S. (1991). Working poor families: Trends, causes, effects, and suggested policies. *Family Relations, 40,* 191-198.

Chilman, C. S. (1993). Parental employment and child care trends: Some critical issues and suggested policies. *Social Work, 38*(4), 451-460.

Christensen, K. E., & Staines, G. L. (1990). Flextime: A viable solution to work/family conflict? *Journal of Family Issues, 11*(4), 455-476.

Clark-Nicolas, P., & Gray-Little, B. (1991). Effect of economic resources on marital quality in black married couples. *Journal of Marriage and the Family, 53,* 645-655.

Cobb, S., & Kasl, S. V. (1977). *Termination: The consequences of job loss* (Report No. 76-1261). Cincinnati, OH: National Institute for Occupational Safety and Health.

Cohen, P., Johnson, J., Lewis, S. A., & Brook, J. S. (1990). Single parenthood and employment: Double jeopardy? In J. Eckenrode & S. Gore (Eds.), *Stress between work and family* (pp. 117-132). New York: Plenum.

Combrinck-Graham, L. (1985). A developmental model for family systems. *Family Process, 24*(2), 139-150.

Conger, R. D., Conger, K. J., Elder, G. H., Jr., Lorenz, F. O., Simons, R. L., & Whitbeck, L. B. (1992). A family process model of economic hardship and adjustment of early adolescent boys. *Child Development, 63,* 526-541.

Conger, R. D., & Elder, G. H., Jr., (1994). *Families in troubled times: Adapting to change in rural America.* Hawthorne, NY: Aldine de Gruyter.

Conger, R. D., Elder, G. H., Jr., Lorenz, F. O., Conger, K. J., Simons, R. L., Whitbeck, L. B., Huck, S., & Melby, J. N. (1990). Linking economic hardship to marital quality and instability. *Journal of Marriage and the Family, 52,* 643-656.

Conger, R. D., Lorenz, F. O., Elder, G. H., Jr., Melby, J. N., Simons, R. L., & Conger, K. J. (1991). A process model of family economic pressure and early adolescent alcohol use. *Journal of Early Adolescence, 11*(4), 430-449.

Corrigan, P. W., MacKain, S. J., & Liberman, R. P. (1994). Skill training modules—A strategy for dissemination and utilization of a rehabilitation innovation. In J. Rothman & E. J. Thomas (Eds.), *Intervention research: Design and development for human service* (pp. 317-352). New York: Haworth.

Coulton, C. J., & Pandey, S. (1992). Geographic concentration of poverty and risk to children in urban neighborhoods. *American Behavioral Scientist, 35*(3), 238-257.

Covin, T. J., & Brush, C. C. (1991). An examination of male and female attitudes toward career and family issues. *Sex Roles, 25,* 393-415.

Crosbie-Burnett, M., & Lewis, E. A. (1993). Use of African-American family structures and functioning to address the challenges of European-American postdivorce families. *Family Relations, 42,* 243-248.

Dail, P. W. (1988). Unemployment and family stress. *Public Welfare, 46*(1), 30-34.

Danziger, S. H., Sandefur, G. D., & Weinberg, D. H. (Eds.). (1994). *Confronting poverty: Prescriptions for change.* Cambridge, MA: Harvard University Press.

Davis, L. E., & Proctor, E. K. (1989). *Race, gender and class: Guidelines for practice with individuals, families, and groups.* Englewood Cliffs, NJ: Prentice Hall.

Devine, J. A., & Wright, J. D. (1993). *The greatest of evils: Urban poverty and the American underclass.* Hawthorne, NY: Aldine de Gruyter.

DiBenedetto, B., & Tittle, C. K. (1990). Gender and adult roles: Role commitment of women and men in a job-family trade-off context. *Journal of Counseling Psychology, 37*(1), 41-48.

Dolgoff, R., Feldstein, D., & Skolnik, L. (1993). *Understanding social welfare* (3rd ed.). New York: Longman.

Donovan, R., Jaffe, N., & Pirie, V. M. (1987). Unemployment among low-income women: An exploratory study. *Social Work, 32,* 301-305.

Dooley, D., & Catalano, R. (1988). Recent research on the psychological effects of unemployment. *Journal of Social Issues, 44*(4), 1-12.

Dore, M. M. (1993). Family preservation and poor families: When "homebuilding" is not enough. *Families in Society, 74*(9), 545-556.

Dunlap, K. M. (1993). A history of research in social work education: 1915-1991. *Journal of Social Work Education, 29*(3), 293-301.

Eckenrode, J., & Gore, S. (Eds.). (1990). *Stress between work and family.* New York: Plenum Press.

Edelman, M. W. (1987). *Families in peril: An agenda for social change.* Cambridge, MA: Harvard University Press.

Elder, G. H., Jr. (1974). *Children of the Great Depression.* Chicago: University of Chicago Press.

Elder, G. H., Jr., & Caspi, A. (1988). Economic stress in lives: Developmental perspectives. *Journal of Social Issues, 44*(4), 25-45.

Elder, G. H., Jr., Conger, R. D., Foster, E. M., & Ardelt, M. (1992). Families under economic pressure. *Journal of Family Issues, 13*(1), 5-37.

Elder, G. H., Jr., & Rockwell, R. C. (1985). Children of hard times: Perspectives from the social change project. In J. Boulet, A. M. Debritto, & S. A. Ray (Eds.), *Understanding the economic crisis: The impact of poverty and unemployment on children and families* (pp. 43-63). Ann Arbor: University of Michigan (Bush Program in Child Development and Social Policy).

Ellman, B., & Taggart, M. (1993). Changing gender norms. In F. Walsh (Ed.), *Normal family processes* (2nd ed., pp. 377-404). New York: Guilford.

Ellwood, D. T. (1988). *Poor support: Poverty in the American family.* New York: Basic Books.

Ellwood, D. T., & Crane, J. (1990). Family change among black Americans: What do we know? *Journal of Economic Perspectives, 4*(4), 65-84.

Ensminger, M. E., & Celentano, D. D. (1990). Gender differences in the effect of unemployment on psychological distress. *Social Science and Medicine, 30*(4), 469-477.

Epstein, N. B., Baldwin, L. M., & Bishop, D. S. (1983). The McMaster Family Assessment Device. *Journal of Marital and Family Therapy, 9*(2), 171-180.

Epstein, N. B., Bishop, D. S., & Baldwin, L. M. (1982). McMaster model of family functioning: A view of the normal family. In F. Walsh (Ed.), *Normal family processes* (pp. 115-141). New York: Guilford.

Ferman, L. A., & Gardner, J. (1979). Economic deprivation, social mobility, and mental health. In L. A. Ferman & J. P. Gordus (Eds.), *Mental health and the economy* (pp. 193-224). Kalamazoo, MI: Upjohn Institute for Employment Research.

Ferman, L. A., & Gordus, J. P. (Eds.). (1979). *Mental health and the economy.* Kalamazoo, MI: Upjohn Institute for Employment Research.

Fiese, B. H., Hooker, K. A., Kotary, L., & Schwagler, J. (1993). Family rituals in the early stages of parenthood. *Journal of Marriage and the Family, 55,* 633-642.

Figley, C. R., & McCubbin, H. I. (Eds.). (1983). *Stress and the family. Vol. 2: Coping with catastrophe.* New York: Brunner/Mazel.

Figueira-McDonough, J. (1978). Mental health among unemployed Detroiters. *Social Service Review, 52,* 383-399.

Fischer, J., & Corcoran, K. (1994). *Measures for clinical practice* (2nd ed.). New York: Free Press.

Flanagan, C. A. (1990). Change in family work status: Effects on parent-adolescent decision making. *Child Development, 61,* 163-177.

Frese, M. (1987). Alleviating depression in the unemployed: Adequate financial support, hope, and early retirement. *Social Science and Medicine, 25*(2), 213-215.

Friedman, D. E. (1986). Painting the child care landscape: A palette of inadequacy and innovation. In S. A. Hewlett, A. S. Ilchman, & J. J. Sweeney (Eds.), *Family and work: Bridging the gap* (pp. 67-89). Cambridge, MA: Ballinger.

Galbraith, J. K. (1992). *The culture of contentment.* New York: Houghton Mifflin.

Galinsky, E., & Stein, P. J. (1990). The impact of human resource policies on employees: Balancing work/family life. *Journal of Family Issues, 11*(4), 368-383.

Ganong, L. H., & Coleman, M. (1987). Effects of parental remarriage on children: An updated comparison of theories, methods, and findings from clinical and empirical research. In K. Pasley & M. Ihinger-Tallman (Eds.), *Remarriage and stepparenting* (pp. 94-140). New York: Guilford.

Garfinkel, I. (1992). Bringing fathers back in: The child support assurance strategy. *The American Prospect, 9,* 74-83.

Garfinkel, I., & McLanahan, S. S. (1986). *Single mothers and their children: A new American dilemma.* Washington, DC: Urban Institute Press.

Garvin, C. D., & Seabury, B. A. (1984). *Interpersonal practice in social work: Processes and procedures.* Englewood Cliffs, NJ: Prentice Hall.

Germain, C. B., & Gitterman, A. (1987). Ecological perspective. In A. Minahan (Ed.), *Encyclopedia of social work* (18th ed., Vol. 1, pp. 488-499). Silver Spring, MD: National Association of Social Workers.

Gerstel, N., & Gallagher, S. K. (1993). Kinkeeping and distress: Gender, recipients of care, and work-family conflict. *Journal of Marriage and the Family, 55,* 598-607.

Gerstel, N., & Gross, H. E. (Eds.). (1987). *Families and work.* Philadelphia, PA: Temple University Press.

Gilbert, N., Specht, H., & Terrell, P. (1993). *Dimensions of social welfare policy* (3rd ed.). Englewood Cliffs, NJ: Prentice Hall.

Ginzberg, E. (1943). *The unemployed.* New York: Harper & Brothers.

Godwin, D. D., Draughn, P. S., Little, L. F., & Marlowe, J. (1991). Wives' off-farm employment, farm family economic status, and family relationships. *Journal of Marriage and the Family, 53,* 389-402.

Goff, S. J., Mount, M. K., & Jamison, R. L. (1990). Employer supported child care, work/family conflict, and absenteeism: A field study. *Personnel Psychology, 43,* 793-809.

Googins, B. K. (1991). *Work/family conflicts: Private lives—public responses.* New York: Auburn House.

Gordus, J. P., Jarley, P., & Ferman, L. A. (1981). *Plant closings and economic dislocation.* Kalamazoo, MI: Upjohn Institute for Employment Research.

Gove, P. B. (Ed.). (1976). *Webster's third new international dictionary of the English language* (Unabridged). Springfield, MA: Merriam.

Graber, H., Haywood, S., & Vosler, N. R. (in press). An empowerment model for building neighborhood community: Grace Hill Neighborhood Services. *Journal of Progressive Human Services.*

Grayson, J. P. (1985). The closure of a factory and its impact on health. *International Journal of Health Services, 15*(1), 69-93.

Grayson, P. (1986). Plant closures and political despair. *Canadian Review of Sociology and Anthropology, 23*(3), 331-349.

Green, G. D., & Bozett, F. W. (1991). Lesbian mothers and gay fathers. In J. C. Gonsiorek & J. D. Weinrich (Eds.), *Homosexuality: Research implications for public policy* (pp. 197-214). Newbury Park, CA: Sage.

Green, R. G., & Vosler, N. R. (1992). Issues in the assessment of family practice: An empirical study. *Journal of Social Service Research, 15*(3/4), 1-19.

Greenstein, T. N. (1990). Marital disruption and the employment of married women. *Journal of Marriage and the Family, 52,* 657-676.

Gueron, J. M., & Pauly, E. (1991). *From welfare to work.* New York: Russell Sage.

Hamermesh, D. S. (1989). What do we know about worker displacement in the U.S.? *Industrial Relations, 28*(1), 51-59.

Hamilton, V. L., Broman, C. L., Hoffman, W. S., & Renner, D. S. (1990, June). Hard times and vulnerable people: Initial effects of plant closing on autoworkers' mental health. *Journal of Health and Social Behavior, 31,* 123-140.

Hamilton, V. L., Hoffman, W. S., Broman, C. L., & Rauma, D. (1993). Unemployment, distress, and coping: A panel study of autoworkers. *Journal of Personality and Social Psychology, 65*(2), 234-247.

Hanks, R. S. (1990). The impact of early retirement incentives on retirees and their families. *Journal of Family Issues, 11,* 424-437.

Hansen, G. B. (1988). Layoffs, plant closings, and worker displacement in America: Serious problems that need a national solution. *Journal of Social Issues, 44*(4), 153-171.

Harley, S. (1990). For the good of family and race: Gender, work, and domestic roles in the black community, 1880-1930. *Signs: Journal of Women in Culture and Society, 15*(2), 336-349.

Hartman, A. (1978). Diagrammatic assessment of family relationships. *Social Casework, 59,* 465-476.

Hartman, A. (1993). Challenges for family policy. In F. Walsh (Ed.), *Normal family processes* (2nd ed., pp. 474-502). New York: Guilford.

Hartman, A. (1995). Ideological themes in family policy. *Families in Society, 76*(3), 182-192.

Hartman, A., & Laird, J. (1983). *Family-centered social work practice.* New York: Free Press.

Hartman, A., & Laird, J. (1987). Family practice. In A. Minahan (Ed.), *Encyclopedia of social work* (18th ed., Vol. 1, pp. 575-589). Silver Spring, MD: National Association of Social Workers.

Hasenfeld, Y., & Furman, W. M. (1994). Intervention research as an interorganizational exchange. In J. Rothman & E. J. Thomas (Eds.), *Intervention research: Design and development for human service* (pp. 297-313). New York: Haworth.

Hesketh, B., Shouksmith, G., & Kang, J. (1987). A case study and balance sheet approach to unemployment. *Journal of Counseling and Development, 66,* 175-179.

Hetherington, E. M., Stanley-Hagan, M., & Anderson, E. R. (1989). Marital transitions: A child's perspective. *American Psychologist, 44,* 303-312.

Hewlett, S. A., Ilchman, A. S., & Sweeney, J. J. (Eds.). (1986). *Family and work: Bridging the gap.* Cambridge, MA: Ballinger.

Higgins, C., Duxbury, L., & Lee, C. (1994). Impact of life-cycle stage and gender on the ability to balance work and family responsibilities. *Family Relations, 43*(2), 144-150.

Hill, R. (1949). *Families under stress.* New York: Harper & Row.

Hill, R. (1958). Generic features of families under stress. *Social Casework, 49,* 139-150.

Hill, R. B. (with Billingsley, A., Engram, E., Malson, M. R., Rubin, R. H., Stack, C. B., Stewart, J. B., & Teele, J. E.). (1993). *Research on the African-American family: A holistic perspective.* Westport, CT: Auburn House.

Hochschild, A. (1989). *The second shift.* New York: Viking.

Hoff, M. D. (1992, July). *Integrating global environmental issues into the social work curriculum.* Paper presented at the 26th International Congress of the International Association of Schools of Social Work, Washington, DC.

Hoff, M. D., & McNutt, J. G. (1994). *The global environmental crisis: Implications for social welfare and social work.* Brookfield, VT: Ashgate.

Hoff, M. D., & Polack, R. J. (1993). Social dimensions of the environmental crisis: Challenges for social work. *Social Work, 38*(2), 204-211.

Hoffman, W. S., Carpentier-Alting, P., Thomas, D., Hamilton, V. L., & Broman, C. L. (1991). Initial impact of plant closings on automobile workers and their families. *Families in Society, 72,* 103-107.

Hoffman, W. S., Hamilton, V. L., Broman, C. L., & Rauma, D. (1991, April). *Aftermath: A panel study of unemployment and mental health among autoworkers.* Paper presented at the North Central Sociological Association, Dearborn, MI.

Holland, T. P., & Kilpatrick, A. C. (1993). Using narrative techniques to enhance multicultural practice. *Journal of Social Work Education, 29*(3), 302-308.

Hollingshead, A. B., & Redlich, F. C. (1958). *Social class and mental illness: A community study.* New York: John Wiley.

Hopps, J. G., Pinderhughes, E., & Shankar, R. (1995). *The power to care: Clinical practice effectiveness with overwhelmed clients.* New York: Free Press.

Howland, M. (1988). *Plant closings and worker displacement: The regional issues.* Kalamazoo, MI: Upjohn Institute for Employment Research.

Howland, M., & Peterson, G. E. (1988). Labor market conditions and the reemployment of displaced workers. *Industrial and Labor Relations Review, 42*(1), 109-122.

Huber, J. (1988). A theory of family, economy, and gender. *Journal of Family Issues, 9*(1), 9-26.

Hudson, W. W. (1982). *The clinical measurement package: A field manual.* Homewood, IL: Dorsey.

Ihinger-Tallman, M. (1986). Member adjustment in single parent families: Theory building. *Family Relations, 35,* 215-221.

Institute of Cultural Affairs. (1981). Analyzing social change: Facing the future by thinking comprehensively. *Image, 11*(1), 8-9.

Iversen, L., & Sabroe, S. (1988). Psychological well-being among unemployed and employed people after a company closedown: A longitudinal study. *Journal of Social Issues, 44*(4), 141-152.

Jackson, P. R., & Walsh, S. (1987). Unemployment and the family. In D. Fryer & P. Ullah (Eds.), *Unemployed people: Social and psychological perspectives* (pp. 194-216). Milton Keynes, UK: Open University Press.

Jansson, B. S. (1994). *Social policy: From theory to policy practice* (2nd ed.). Pacific Grove, CA: Brooks/Cole.

Janzen, C., & Harris, O. (1986). *Family treatment in social work practice* (2nd ed.). Itasca, IL: Peacock.

Joelson, L., & Wahlquist, L. (1987). The psychological meaning of job insecurity and job loss: Results of a longitudinal study. *Social Science and Medicine, 25*(2), 179-182.

Johnson, D. R., & Booth, A. (1990). Rural economic decline and marital quality: A panel study of farm marriages. *Family Relations, 39,* 159-165.

Jones, L. (1988). Unemployment and social integration: A review. *Journal of Sociology and Social Welfare, 15*(4), 161-176.

Jones, L. (1989). Effect of unemployment on women. *Affilia, 4*(4), 54-67.

Jones, L. (1990). Unemployment and child abuse. *Families in Society, 71*(10), 579-586.

Jones, L. (1991a). Unemployed fathers and their children: Implications for policy and practice. *Child and Adolescent Social Work, 8*(2), 101-116.

Jones, L. (1991b). Unemployment: The effect of social networks, depression, and reemployment opportunities. *Journal of Social Service Research, 15*(1/2), 1-22.

Kagan, A. R. (1987). Unemployment causes ill health: The wrong track. *Social Science and Medicine, 25*(2), 217-218.

Kalleberg, A. L., & Rosenfeld, R. A. (1990). Work in the family and in the labor market: A cross-national, reciprocal analysis. *Journal of Marriage and the Family, 52,* 331-346.

Kamerman, S. B. (1986). Maternity, paternity, and parenting policies: How does the United States compare? In S. A. Hewlett, A. S. Ilchman, & J. J. Sweeney (Eds.), *Family and work: Bridging the gap* (pp. 53-65). Cambridge, MA: Ballinger.

Kamerman, S. B., & Kahn, A. J. (1981). *Child care, family benefits, and working parents.* New York: Columbia University Press.

Kanter, R. M. (1977). *Work and family in the United States: A critical review and agenda for research and policy.* New York: Russell Sage.

Kasl, S. V., & Cobb, S. (1970). Blood pressure changes in men undergoing job loss: A preliminary report. *Psychosomatic Medicine, 32*(1), 19-38.

Kasl, S. V., Gore, S., & Cobb, S. (1975). The experience of losing a job: Reported changes in health, symptoms and illness behavior. *Psychosomatic Medicine, 37*(2), 106-122.

Kelly, R. F., & Voydanoff, P. (1985). Work/family role strain among employed parents. *Family Relations, 34,* 367-374.

Kessler, R. C., Turner, J. B., & House, J. S. (1987). Intervening processes in the relationship between unemployment and health. *Psychological Medicine, 17,* 949-961.

Kessler, R. C., Turner, J. B., & House, J. S. (1988). Effects of unemployment on health in a community survey: Main, modifying, and mediating effects. *Journal of Social Issues, 44*(4), 69-85.

Kessler, R. C., Turner, J. B., & House, J. S. (1989). Unemployment, reemployment, and emotional functioning in a community sample. *American Sociological Review, 54,* 648-657.

Kissman, K. (1990). Women in blue-collar occupations: An exploration of constraints and facilitators. *Journal of Sociology and Social Welfare, 17*(3), 139-149.

Klein, W. C., & Bloom, M. (1994). Social work as applied social science: A historical analysis. *Social Work, 39*(4), 421-431.

Kolevzon, M. S., & Green, R. G. (1985). *Family therapy models: Convergence and divergence.* New York: Springer.

Kolevzon, M. S., Green, R. G., Fortune, A. E., & Vosler, N. R. (1988). Evaluating family therapy: Divergent methods, divergent findings. *Journal of Marital and Family Therapy, 14*(3), 277-286.

Komarovsky, M. (1940). *The unemployed man and his family: The effect of unemployment upon the status of the man in fifty-nine families.* New York: Dryden.

Korsching, P. F., & Lasley, P. (1990). Problems with the official unemployment rate as the distribution basis of federal assistance in rural areas. *Human Services in the Rural Environment, 13*(3), 21-26.

Krystal, E., Moran-Sackett, M., Thompson, S. V., & Cantoni, L. (1983). Serving the unemployed. *Social Casework, 64,* 67-76.

Laird, J. (1984). Sorcerers, shamans, and social workers: The use of ritual in social work practice. *Social Work, 29*(2), 123-129.

Laird, J. (1993). Lesbian and gay families. In F. Walsh (Ed.), *Normal family processes* (2nd ed., pp. 282-328). New York: Guilford.

Lamb, M. E. (1987). Introduction: The emergent American father. In M. E. Lamb (Ed.), *The father's role: Cross-cultural perspectives* (pp. 3-25). Hillsdale, NJ: Lawrence Erlbaum.

Lambert, S. J. (1993). Workplace policies as social policy. *Social Service Review, 67*(2), 237-260.

Larson, J. H., Wilson, S. M., & Beley, R. (1994). The impact of job insecurity on marital and family relationships. *Family Relations, 43,* 138-143.

Lazarus, R. S., & Folkman, S. (1984). *Stress, appraisal, and coping.* New York: Springer.

Leira, A. (1992). *Welfare states and working mothers: The Scandinavian experience.* Cambridge, UK: Cambridge University Press.

Levitan, S. R., & Gallo, F. (1993). *Jobs for JOBS: Toward a work-based welfare system.* Washington, DC: Center for Social Policy Studies.

Levy, F. S., & Michel, R. C. (1991). *The economic future of American families: Income and wealth trends.* Washington, DC: Urban Institute Press.

Lewis, J. M., Beavers, W. R., Gossett, J. T., & Phillips, V. A. (1976). *No single thread: Psychological health in family systems.* New York: Brunner/Mazel.

Lewis, J. M., & Looney, J. G. (1983). *The long struggle: Well-functioning working-class black families.* New York: Brunner/Mazel.

Lewis, S. (1992, July). *The world of our children: What will it be?* Paper presented at the World Assembly of the National Association of Social Workers and the International Federation of Social Workers, Washington, DC.

Liem, R. (1985). Unemployment: A family as well as a personal crisis. In J. Boulet, A. M. Debritto, & S. A. Ray (Eds.), *Understanding the economic crisis: The impact of poverty and unemployment on children and families* (pp. 112-118). Ann Arbor, MI: University of Michigan (Bush Program in Child Development and Social Policy).

Liem, R., & Liem, J. H. (1988). Psychological effects of unemployment on workers and their families. *Journal of Social Issues, 44*(4), 87-105.

Liem, R., & Rayman, P. (1982). Health and social costs of unemployment: Research and policy considerations. *American Psychologist, 37*(10), 1116-1123.

Lightburn, A., & Kemp, S. P. (1994). Family-support programs: Opportunities for community-based practice. *Families in Society, 75*(1), 16-26.

Liker, J. K., & Elder, G. H., Jr. (1983). Economic hardship and marital relations in the 1930s. *American Sociological Review, 48,* 343-359.

Macklin, E. D. (1980). Nontraditional family forms: A decade of research. In F. M. Berardo (Ed.), *Decade review: Family research 1970-1979* (pp. 175-192). Minneapolis, MN: National Council on Family Relations. [Also published as a special issue of *Journal of Marriage and the Family,* 1980, *42*(4)]

Madden, J. F. (1988). The distribution of economic losses among displaced workers: Measurement methods matter. *Journal of Human Resources, 23*(1), 93-107.

Main, M., & Goldwyn, R. (1984). Predicting rejection of her infant from mother's representation of her own experience: Implications for the abused-abusing intergenerational cycle. *Child Abuse & Neglect, 8,* 203-217.

Main, M., Kaplan, N., & Cassidy, U. (1985). Security of attachment in infancy, childhood, and adulthood: A move to the level of representation. In I. Bretherton & E. Waters (Ed.), *Growing points of attachment theory and research* (pp. 66-104). Monographs of the Society for Research in Child Development, Serial No. 209(1-2).

Mancini, J. A., & Blieszner, R. (1991). Aging parents and adult children: Research themes in intergenerational relations. In A. Booth (Ed.), *Contemporary families: Looking forward, looking back* (pp. 248-264). Minneapolis, MN: National Council on Family Relations.

Marger, M. N. (1991). *Race and ethnic relations: American and global perspectives* (2nd ed.). Belmont, CA: Wadsworth.

Marlow, C. (1991). Women, children and employment: Responses by the United States and Great Britain. *International Social Work, 34,* 287-297.

Martin, J. M., & Martin, E. P. (1985). *The helping tradition in the black family and community.* Silver Spring, MD: National Association of Social Workers.

Mattaini, M. A. (1993). *More than a thousand words: Graphics for clinical practice.* Washington, DC: NASW Press.

McAdoo, H. P. (1982). Levels of stress and family support in black families. In H. I. McCubbin, A. E. Cauble, & J. M. Patterson (Eds.), *Family stress, coping, and social support* (pp. 239-252). Springfield, IL: Charles C Thomas.

McAdoo, H. P. (1993). It takes a whole village to raise a child. *Family Resource Coalition Report, 12*(1), 14-15.

McCubbin, H. I., & Figley, C. R. (1983). *Stress and the family. Vol. 1: Coping with normative transitions.* New York: Brunner/Mazel.

McCubbin, H. I., Joy, C. B., Cauble, A. E., Comeau, J. K., Patterson, J. M., & Needle, R. H. (1980). Family stress and coping: A decade review. In F. M. Berardo (Ed.), *Decade review: Family research 1970-1979* (pp. 125-141). Minneapolis, MN: National Council on Family Relations. [Also published as a special issue of *Journal of Marriage and the Family,* 1980, *42*(4)]

McCubbin, H. I., Nevin, R. S., Cauble, A. E., Larsen, A., Comeau, J. K., & Patterson, J. M. (1982). Family coping with chronic illness: The case of cerebral palsy. In H. I. McCubbin, A. E. Cauble, & J. M. Patterson (Eds.), *Family stress, coping, and social support* (pp. 169-188). Springfield, IL: Charles C Thomas.

McCubbin, H. I., & Patterson, J. M. (1983). The family stress process: The double ABCX model of adjustment and adaptation. In H. I. McCubbin, M. B. Sussman, & J. M. Patterson (Eds.), *Social stress and the family: Advances and developments in family stress theory and research* (pp. 7-37). New York: Haworth.

McGoldrick, M. (1993). Ethnicity, cultural diversity, and normality. In F. Walsh (Ed.), *Normal family processes* (2nd ed., pp. 331-360). New York: Guilford.

McGoldrick, M., & Gerson, R. (1985). *Genograms in family assessment.* New York: Norton.

McGoldrick, M., Heiman, M., & Carter, B. (1993). The changing family life cycle: A perspective on normalcy. In F. Walsh (Ed.), *Normal family processes* (2nd ed., pp. 405-443). New York: Guilford.

McGoldrick, M., Pearce, J. K., & Giordano, J. (1982). *Ethnicity and family therapy.* New York: Guilford.

McInnis-Dittrich, K. (1994). *Integrating social welfare policy and social work practice.* Pacific Grove, CA: Brooks/Cole.

McLanahan, S., & Booth, K. (1991). Mother-only families: Problems, prospects, and politics. In A. Booth (Ed.), *Contemporary families: Looking forward, looking back* (pp. 405-428). Minneapolis, MN: National Council on Family Relations.

McLeod, J. D., & Kessler, R. C. (1990, June). Socioeconomic status differences in vulnerability to undesirable life events. *Journal of Health and Social Behavior, 31,* 162-172.

McLoyd, V. C. (1990). The impact of economic hardship on black families and children: Psychological distress, parenting, and socioemotional development. *Child Development, 61,* 311-346.

McLoyd, V. C., & Wilson, L. (1990). Maternal behavior, social support, and economic conditions as predictors of distress in children. In V. C. McLoyd & C. A. Flanagan (Eds.), *Economic stress: Effects on family life and child development* (pp. 49-69). San Francisco: Jossey-Bass.

Mederer, H., & Hill, R. (1983). Critical transitions over the family life span: Theory and research. In H. I. McCubbin, M. B. Sussman, & J. M. Patterson (Eds.), *Social stress and the family: Advances and developments in family stress theory and research* (pp. 39-60). New York: Haworth.

Mederer, H. J. (1993). Division of labor in two-earner homes: Task accomplishment versus household management as critical variables in perceptions about family work. *Journal of Marriage and the Family, 55,* 133-145.

Menaghan, E. G., & Parcel, T. L. (1991). Parental employment and family life: Research in the 1980s. In A. Booth (Ed.), *Contemporary families: Looking forward, looking back* (pp. 361-380). Minneapolis, MN: National Council on Family Relations.

Meyer, C. H. (1976). *Social work practice* (2nd ed.). New York: Free Press.

Meyer, C. H. (Ed.). (1983). *Clinical social work in the eco-systems perspective.* New York: Columbia University Press.

Meyers, M. K. (1990). The ABCs of child care in a mixed economy: A comparison of public and private sector alternatives. *Social Service Review, 64*(4), 559-579.

Meyers, S. A. (1993). Adapting parent education programs to meet the needs of fathers: An ecological perspective. *Family Relations, 42,* 447-452.

Miller, B. (1987). Counseling gay husbands and fathers. In F. W. Bozett (Ed.), *Gay and lesbian parents* (pp. 175-187). New York: Praeger.

Miller, M. L., Moen, P., & Dempster-McClain, D. (1991). Motherhood, multiple roles, and maternal well-being: Women of the 1950s. *Gender & Society, 5*(4), 565-582.

Mincy, R. B. (1990). Raising the minimum wage: Effects on family poverty. *Monthly Labor Review, 113*(7), 18-25.

Minuchin, S. (1974). *Families and family therapy.* Cambridge, MA: Harvard University Press.

Mirowsky, J., & Ross, C. E. (1989). *Social causes of psychological distress.* Hawthorne, NY: Aldine de Gruyter.

Moen, P. (1982). Preventing financial hardship: Coping strategies of families of the unemployed. In H. I. McCubbin, A. E. Cauble, & J. M. Patterson (Eds.), *Family stress, coping, and social support* (pp. 151-168). Springfield, IL: Charles C Thomas.

Moen, P. (1989). *Working parents: Transformations in gender roles and public policies in Sweden.* Madison, WI: University of Wisconsin Press.

Moen, P. (1992). *Women's two roles: A contemporary dilemma.* New York: Auburn House.

Moos, R. H., & Moos, B. S. (1986). *Family Environment Scale manual* (2nd ed.). Palo Alto, CA: Consulting Psychologists Press.

Mulroy, E. (1990). Single-parent families and the housing crisis: Implications for macro-practice. *Social Work, 35*(6), 542-546.

Nair, S., Blake, M. L., & Vosler, N. R. (1993). *Ang Mo Kio Family Service Centres Research Forms.* Singapore: Ang Mo Kio Social Service Centre.

Nair, S., Blake, M. L., & Vosler, N. R. (in press). Multilevel social systems practice with low income families in Singapore: A pilot study of key factors. *Families in Society.*

National Association of Social Workers. (1982). Changes in NASW family policy. *NASW News, 27*(2), 10.

National Association of Social Workers. (1993). *NASW code of ethics.* Washington, DC: National Association of Social Workers, Inc.

Nelson, K. E., Saunders, E. J., & Landsman, M. J. (1993). Chronic child neglect in perspective. *Social Work, 38*(6), 661-671.

Newman, K. S. (1993). *Declining fortunes: The withering of the American dream.* New York: Basic Books.

Nurius, P. S., & Hudson, W. W. (1993). *Human services practice, evaluation, and computers: A practical guide for today and beyond.* Pacific Grove, CA: Brooks/Cole.

Olson, D. H. (1986). Circumplex Model VII: Validation studies and FACES III. *Family Process, 25,* 337-351.

Olson, D. H. (1993). Circumplex Model of marital and family systems: Assessing family functioning. In F. Walsh (Ed.), *Normal family processes* (2nd ed., pp. 104-137). New York: Guilford.

Olson, D. H., & Lavee, Y. (1989). Family systems and family stress: A family life cycle perspective. In K. Kreppner & R. M. Lerner (Eds.), *Family systems and life-span development* (pp. 165-195). Hillsdale, NJ: Lawrence Erlbaum.

Olson, D. H., McCubbin, H. I., Barnes, H., Larsen, A., Muxen, M., & Wilson, M. (1983). *Families: What makes them work.* Beverly Hills, CA: Sage.

Olson, D. H., Sprenkle, D. H., & Russell, C. S. (1979). Circumplex Model of marital and family systems I: Cohesion and adaptability dimensions, family types, and clinical applications. *Family Process, 18,* 3-28.

Ozawa, M. N. (1982). *Income maintenance and work incentives: Toward a synthesis.* New York: Praeger.

Ozawa, M. N. (Ed.). (1989). *Women's life cycle and economic insecurity: Problems and proposals.* New York: Praeger.

Ozawa, M. N. (1991). Basis of income support for children: A time for change. *Children and Youth Services Review, 13,* 7-27.

Ozawa, M. N., & Wang, Y. T. (1993). Can AFDC families be economically self-sufficient? *New England Journal of Human Services, 12*(1), 19-26.

Papp, P. (Writer, Narrator, & Therapist), Charles, B., & Walker, G. (Producers & Editors). (1974). *Making the invisible visible* [Clinical Training Videotape]. New York: Ackerman Institute for Family Therapy.

Parsons, T., & Bales, R. F. (1955). *Family, socialization and interaction process.* New York: Free Press.

Pearlin, L. I., & Turner, H. A. (1987). The family as a context of the stress process. In S. V. Kasl & C. L. Cooper (Eds.), *Stress and health: Issues in research methodology* (pp. 143-165). New York: John Wiley.

Perrucci, C. C., Perrucci, R., Targ, D. B., & Targ, H. R. (1985). Impact of a plant closing on workers and the community. In R. L. Simpson & I. H. Simpson (Eds.), *Research in the sociology of work: A research annual* (Vol. 3: *Unemployment,* pp. 231-260). Greenwich, CT: JAI.

Perrucci, C. C., Perrucci, R., Targ, D. B., & Targ, H. R. (1988). *Plant closings: International context and social costs.* Hawthorne, NY: Aldine de Gruyter.

Pies, C. (1987). Considering parenthood: Psychosocial issues for gay men and lesbians choosing alternative fertilization. In F. W. Bozett (Ed.), *Gay and lesbian parents* (pp. 165-174). New York: Praeger.

Piotrkowski, C. S., & Hughes, D. (1993). Dual-earner families in context: Managing family and work systems. In F. Walsh (Ed.), *Normal family process* (2nd ed., pp. 185-207). New York: Guilford.

Piotrkowski, C. S., Rapoport, R., & Rapoport, R. (1987). Families and work. In M. B. Sussman & S. K. Steinmetz (Eds.), *Handbook of marriage and the family* (pp. 251-283). New York: Plenum.

Pleck, J. H. (1985). *Working wives/working husbands.* Beverly Hills, CA: Sage.

Pleck, J. H., & Staines, G. L. (1985). Work schedules and family life in two-earner couples. *Journal of Family Issues, 6,* 61-82.

Podgursky, M., & Swaim, P. (1987). Health insurance loss: The case of the displaced worker. *Monthly Labor Review, 110*(4), 30-33.

Popenoe, D. (1993). American family decline, 1960-1990: A review and appraisal. *Journal of Marriage and the Family, 55,* 527-555.

Pottick, K. J. (1989). The work role as a major life role. *Social Casework, 70,* 488-494.

Proctor, E. K., Davis, L. E., & Vosler, N. R. (1995). Families: Direct practice. In R. L. Edwards (Ed.-in-Chief), *Encyclopedia of Social Work* (19th ed., Vol. 2, pp. 941-950). Washington, DC: NASW Press.

Raabe, P. H. (1990). The organizational effects of workplace family policies: Past weaknesses and recent progress toward improved research. *Journal of Family Issues, 11*(4), 477-491.

Rank, M. R. (1994). *Living on the edge: The realities of welfare in America.* New York: Columbia University Press.

Richmond, M. E. (1917). *Social diagnosis.* New York: Russell Sage.

Robertson, E. B., Elder, G. H., Jr., Skinner, M. L., & Conger, R. D. (1991). The costs and benefits of social support in families. *Journal of Marriage and the Family, 53,* 403-416.

Rocha, C. J. (1994). Effects of poverty on working families: Comparing models of stress by race and class (Doctoral dissertation, Washington University, 1994). *Dissertation Abstracts International, 55*(11A), 3644.

Rodgers, H. R., Jr. (1990). *Poor women, poor families: The economic plight of America's female-headed households* (Rev. ed.). Armonk, NY: Sharpe.

Rogge, M. E. (1993). Social work, disenfranchised communities, and the natural environment: Field education opportunities. *Journal of Social Work Education, 29*(1), 111-120.

Rolland, J. S. (1993). Mastering family challenges in serious illness and disability. In F. Walsh (Ed.), *Normal family processes* (2nd ed., pp. 444-473). New York: Guilford.

Rook, K., Dooley, D., & Catalano, R. (1991). Stress transmission: The effects of husbands' job stressors on the emotional health of their wives. *Journal of Marriage and the Family, 53,* 165-177.

Ross, C. E., Mirowsky, J., & Goldsteen, K. (1990). The impact of the family on health: The decade in review. *Journal of Marriage and the Family, 52,* 1059-1078.

Rothman, J., Damron-Rodriguez, J., & Shenassa, E. (1994). Systematic research synthesis —Conceptual integration methods of meta-analysis. In J. Rothman & E. J. Thomas (Eds.), *Intervention research: Design and development for human service* (pp. 133-160). New York: Haworth.

Rothman, J., Teresa, J. G., & Erlich, J. L. (1994). Appendix A: Fostering participation and promoting innovation—Handbook for human service professionals. In J. Rothman & E. J. Thomas (Eds.), *Intervention research: Design and development for human service* (pp. 377-426). New York: Haworth.

Rothman, J., & Thomas, E. J. (Eds.). (1994). *Intervention research: Design and development for human service.* New York: Haworth.

Rubin, A., & Babbie, E. (1993). *Research methods for social work* (2nd ed.). Pacific Grove, CA: Brooks/Cole.

Rubin, L. B. (1976). *Worlds of pain: Life in the working-class family.* New York: Basic Books.

Ruggles, P. (1990). *Drawing the line: Alternative poverty measures and their implications for public policy.* Washington, DC: Urban Institute Press.

Satir, V. (1964). *Conjoint family therapy.* Palo Alto, CA: Science and Behavior Books.

Satir, V. (1983). *Conjoint family therapy* (3rd ed.). Palo Alto, CA: Science and Behavior Books.

Satir, V. (1988). *The new peoplemaking.* Mountain View, CA: Science and Behavior Books.

Schiller, B. R. (1989). *The economics of poverty and discrimination* (5th ed.). Englewood Cliffs, NJ: Prentice Hall.

Schneewind, K. A. (1989). Contextual approaches to family systems research: The macro-micro puzzle. In K. Kreppner & R. M. Lerner (Eds.), *Family systems and life-span development* (pp. 197-221). Hillsdale, NJ: Lawrence Erlbaum.

Schorr, L. B. (with Schorr, D.). (1988). *Within our reach: Breaking the cycle of disadvantage.* New York: Anchor/Doubleday.

Schwartz, M. A., & Scott, B. M. (1994). *Marriages and families: Diversity and change.* Englewood Cliffs, NJ: Prentice Hall.

Segal, E. A. (1991). The juvenilization of poverty in the 1980s. *Social Work, 36*(5), 454-457.

Shapiro, I., & Greenstein, R. (1993). *Making work pay: The unfinished agenda.* Washington, DC: Center on Budget and Policy Priorities.

Sherraden, M. (1985a). Chronic unemployment: A social work perspective. *Social Work, 30,* 403-408.

Sherraden, M. (1985b). Employment policy: A conceptual framework. *Journal of Social Work Education, 21*(2), 5-14.

Sherraden, M. (1991). *Assets and the poor: A new American welfare policy.* Armonk, NY: Sharpe.

Simon, B. L. (1990). Impact of shift work on individuals and families. *Families in Society, 71,* 342-348.

Simons, R. L., Beaman, J., Conger, R. D., & Chao, W. (1993). Stress, support, and antisocial behavior trait as determinants of emotional well-being and parenting practices among single mothers. *Journal of Marriage and the Family, 55,* 385-398.

Skinner, D. A. (1982). The stressors and coping patterns of dual-career families. In H. I. McCubbin, A. E. Cauble, & J. M. Patterson (Eds.), *Family stress, coping, and social support* (pp. 136-150). Springfield, IL: Charles C Thomas.

Smith, R. (1987). *Unemployment and health: A disaster and a challenge.* Oxford, UK: Oxford University Press.

Solomon, B. (1976). *Black empowerment: Social work in oppressed communities.* New York: Columbia University Press.

Spitze, G. (1991). Women's employment and family relations: A review. In A. Booth (Ed.), *Contemporary families: Looking forward, looking back* (pp. 381-404). Minneapolis, MN: National Council on Family Relations.

Staples, R., & Mirande, A. (1980). Racial and cultural variations among American families: A decennial review of the literature on minority families. In F. M. Berardo (Ed.), *Decade review: Family research 1970-1979* (pp. 157-173). Minneapolis, MN: National Council on Family Relations. [Also published as a special issue of *Journal of Marriage and the Family,* 1980, *42*(4)]

Staudohar, P. D., & Brown, H. E. (Eds.). (1987). *Deindustrialization and plant closure.* Lexington, MA: Lexington Books.

Sunley, R., & Sheek, G. W. (1986). *Serving the unemployed and their families.* Milwaukee, WI: Family Service America.

Swiss, D. J., & Walker, J. P. (1993). *Women and the work/family dilemma: How today's professional women are finding solutions.* New York: John Wiley.

Targ, D. B., & Perrucci, C. C. (1990). Plant closings, unemployment and families. *Marriage and Family Review, 15*(3/4), 131-145.

Taylor, R. J., Chatters, L. M., Tucker, M. B., & Lewis, E. (1991). Developments in research on black families: A decade review. In A. Booth (Ed.), *Contemporary families: Looking forward, looking back* (pp. 275-296). Minneapolis, MN: National Council on Family Relations.

Taynor, J., Nelson, R. W., & Daugherty, W. K. (1990). The Family Intervention Scale: Assessing treatment outcome. *Families in Society, 71,* 202-210.

Thoits, P. A. (1983). Dimensions of life events that influence psychological distress. In H. B. Kaplan (Ed.), *Psychosocial stress: Trends in theory and research* (pp. 33-103). New York: Academic Press.

Thomas, V., & Olson, D. H. (1993). Problem families and the Circumplex Model: Observational assessment using the Clinical Rating Scale (CRS). *Journal of Marital and Family Therapy, 19,* 159-175.

Thompson, L. (1991). Family work: Women's sense of fairness. *Journal of Family Issues, 12,* 181-196.

Thompson, L., & Walker, A. J. (1991). Gender in families: Women and men in marriage, work, and parenthood. In A. Booth (Ed.), *Contemporary families: Looking forward, looking back* (pp. 76-102). Minneapolis, MN: National Council on Family Relations.

Touliatos, J., Perlmutter, B. F., & Straus, M. A. (Eds.). (1990). *Handbook of family measurement techniques.* Newbury Park, CA: Sage.

Turner, J. B., Kessler, R. C., & House, J. S. (1991). Factors facilitating adjustment to unemployment: Implications for intervention. *American Journal of Community Psychology, 19*(4), 521-542.

Unger, S. (Ed.). (1977). *The destruction of American Indian families.* New York: Association on American Indian Affairs.

U.S. Bureau of the Census. (1989). *Spells of job search and layoff . . . and their outcomes* (Current Population Reports, Series P-70, No. 16-RD-2). Washington, DC: Government Printing Office.

U.S. Department of Health and Human Services. (1995). The 1995 federal poverty guidelines. *Social Security Bulletin, 58*(1), 87.

Van Hook, M. (1990). Family response to the farm crisis: A study in coping. *Social Work, 35*(5), 425-431.

Vega, W. A. (1991). Hispanic families in the 1980s: A decade of research. In A. Booth (Ed.), *Contemporary families: Looking forward, looking back* (pp. 297-306). Minneapolis, MN: National Council on Family Relations.

Vosler, N. R. (1989). A systems model for child protective services. *Journal of Social Work Education, 25*(1), 20-28.

Vosler, N. R. (1990). Assessing family access to basic resources: An essential component of social work practice. *Social Work, 35,* 434-441.

Vosler, N. R. (1994). Displaced manufacturing workers and their families: A research-based practice model. *Families in Society, 75*(2), 105-115.

Vosler, N. R., & Nair, S. (1993). Families, children, poverty: Education for social work practice at multiple systems levels. *International Social Work, 36,* 159-172.

Vosler, N. R., & Ozawa, M. N. (1992). A multilevel social systems practice model for working with AFDC JOBS program clients. *Families in Society, 73,* 3-12.

Vosler, N. R., & Proctor, E. K. (1990). Stress and competence as predictors of child behavior problems. *Social Work Research and Abstracts, 26*(2), 3-9.

Vosler, N. R., & Proctor, E. K. (1991). Family structure and stressors in a child guidance clinic population. *Families in Society, 72,* 164-173.

Voydanoff, P. (1983). Unemployment: Family strategies for adaptation. In C. R. Figley & H. I. McCubbin (Eds.), *Stress and the family. Vol. 2: Coping with catastrophe* (pp. 90-102). New York: Brunner/Mazel.

Voydanoff, P. (1987). *Work and family life.* Newbury Park, CA: Sage.

Voydanoff, P. (1988). Work and family: A review and expanded conceptualization. In E. B. Goldsmith (Ed.), *Work and family: Theory, research and applications* (pp. 1-22). Corte Madera, CA: Select Press. [Also published as a special issue of *Journal of Social Behavior and Personality,* 1988, *3*(4), 1-22]

Voydanoff, P. (1991). Economic distress and family relations: A review of the eighties. In A. Booth (Ed.), *Contemporary families: Looking forward, looking back* (pp. 429-445). Minneapolis, MN: National Council on Family Relations.

Voydanoff, P., & Donnelly, B. W. (1988). Economic distress, family coping, and quality of family life. In P. Voydanoff & L. C. Majka (Eds.), *Families and economic distress: Coping strategies and social policy* (pp. 97-116). Newbury Park, CA: Sage.

Wagner, D. (1991). Social work and the hidden victims of deindustrialization. *Journal of Progressive Human Services, 2*(1), 15-37.

Waldegrave, C. (1990). Just therapy. *Dulwich Centre Newsletter, 1990*(1), 5-46. (Adelaide, Australia: Dulwich Centre Publications)

Wallace, M., & Rothschild, J. (1988). Plant closings, capital flight, and worker dislocation: The long shadow of deindustrialization. In M. Wallace & J. Rothschild (Eds.), *Research in politics and society* (Vol. 3, pp. 1-35). Greenwich, CT: JAI.

Walsh, F. (1982). Conceptualizations of normal family functioning. In F. Walsh (Ed.), *Normal family processes* (pp. 3-42). New York: Guilford.

Walsh, F. (Ed.). (1993). *Normal family processes* (2nd ed.). New York: Guilford.

Warr, P. (1987). *Work, unemployment, and mental health.* Oxford, UK: Clarendon.

Whitbeck, L. B., Simons, R. L., Conger, R. D., Lorenz, F. O., Huck, S., & Elder, G. H., Jr. (1991). Family economic hardship, parental support, and adolescent self-esteem. *Social Psychology Quarterly, 54*(4), 353-363.

White, M., & Epston, D. (1990). *Narrative means to therapeutic ends.* New York: Norton.

Wicker, A. W., & Burley, K. A. (1991). Close coupling in work-family relationships: Making and implementing decisions in a new family business and at home. *Human Relations, 44*(1), 77-92.

Wilkie, J. R. (1991). The decline in men's labor force participation and income and the changing structure of family economic support. *Journal of Marriage and the Family, 53,* 111-122.

Wilson, W. J. (1987). *The truly disadvantaged: The inner city, the underclass, and public policy.* Chicago: University of Chicago Press.

Winnick, A. J. (1988). The changing distribution of income and wealth in the United States, 1960-1985: An examination of the movement toward two societies, "separate and unequal." In P. Voydanoff & L. C. Majka (Eds.), *Families and economic distress: Coping strategies and social policy* (pp. 232-260). Newbury Park, CA: Sage.

Zimbalist, S. E. (1977). Recent British and American poverty trends: Conceptual and policy contrasts. *Social Service Review, 51*(3), 419-433.

Zimmerman, S. L. (1988). *Understanding family policy: Theoretical approaches.* Newbury Park, CA: Sage.

Zimmerman, S. L. (1992). *Family policies and family well-being: The role of political culture.* Newbury Park, CA: Sage.

Zimmerman, S. L., & Chilman, C. S. (1988). Poverty and families. In C. S. Chilman, F. M. Cox, & E. W. Nunnally (Eds.), *Employment and economic problems* (pp. 107-123). Newbury Park, CA: Sage.

Zippay, A. (1991). Job-training and relocation experiences among displaced industrial workers. *Evaluation Review, 15*(5), 555-570.

Index

ABOUT THE AUTHOR

NANCY R. VOSLER, MSW, LCSW, PhD, is Associate Professor of Social Work in The George Warren Brown School of Social Work at Washington University in St. Louis, Missouri. Her direct practice experience has focused on child and family welfare, and on community-based services. Her research and publications are in the areas of family systems, support programs, family stress and coping, single-parent households and welfare, unemployment, and poverty. She teaches social policy and family practice courses at Washington University, and also has taught at the National University of Singapore, Longwood College, Virginia Commonwealth University, and Northeastern (Oklahoma) State University. In addition, she has supervised social work students for the University of Queensland (Australia) Department of Social Work. She recently taught staff of Family Service Centres in a Diploma Course entitled "A Systems Approach to Marital and Family Counselling"; the course is offered by the Family Resource and Training Centre, a project developed by the Singapore Association of Social Workers.

Dr. Vosler is collaborating with staff of The Ang Mo Kio Family Service Centres to study effective family-focused social work practice with low-income families in Singapore. In the United States, her current research interest is nonmarital coparenting, and the development and evaluation of services for nonmarital parents and their children.

Among her recent publications, she coauthored with Drs. Enola K. Proctor and Larry E. Davis, "Families: Direct Practice," in the 19th edition (1995) of the *Encyclopedia of Social Work* (Washington, DC: NASW Press).